DEATH AND LIFE
IN THE BOXING RING

DOG
ROUNDS

ELLIOT WORSELL

BLINK
bringing you closer

Published by Blink Publishing
3.08, The Plaza,
535 Kings Road,
Chelsea Harbour,
London, SW10 0SZ

www.blinkpublishing.co.uk

facebook.com/blinkpublishing
twitter.com/blinkpublishing

Hardback – 978-1-911274-79-7
Ebook – 978-1-911600-10-7
Paperback – 978-1-788700-25-2

A CIP catalogue of this book is available from the British Library.

Designed by www.envydesign.co.uk
Printed and bound by Clays Ltd, St Ives Plc

1 3 5 7 9 10 8 6 4 2

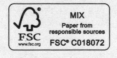

Blink Publishing is an imprint of the Bonnier Publishing Group
www.bonnierpublishing.co.uk

For Nick

CONTENTS

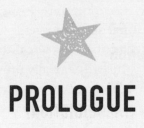

PROLOGUE

The man whose fists put my friend in a coma is behind a closed bathroom door. He's out of reach, out of sight, hiding. In any other scenario, in any other walk of life, the door would be off its hinges and he'd be chased down and reprimanded. There'd be retribution. He'd be brought to justice. But not tonight. Tonight, he will instead be left alone and then comforted. His handiwork will be celebrated. There will be high-fives from those around him, recollections of victory, marks out of ten for his performance. He will receive a championship belt. His father will tell him how proud he is.

This is boxing, the noble art. This is boxing, one of the few domains in which a human being can legally kill another human being. It's for this reason I am in this man's changing room, not in the name of revenge but as witness for the defence, part of this very code. It's why I behave the same as everyone else. I congratulate the winning team and I commiserate the losing one. I discuss and assess the fight as if it is any other sporting event: well, he could have done this or done that; that was a real turning point; what bravery, what heart; the winner really proved himself, didn't he? Acting normal, in boxing terms, is waiting in the victor's changing room rather than hurtling to the hospital or calling the police. This, I'm told, is the process. It's what happens on nights like this when the fight fraternity rallies in the face of looming tragedy and attempts to rationalise something that all of a sudden seems wholly irrational. Besides, the other changing room, the one that belonged to the boxer now in a coma, is cold and empty, eerily so. What use would I be in there? The damage is done.

There's another reason I lurk in the changing room of the man whose fists have put my friend in a coma. This reason, though, has less to do with protocol and more to do with the fact the boxer's father, Chris Eubank, is an invaluable source of knowledge and comfort right now. He has experienced what many of us are experiencing for the first time: the hurt, the confusion, the guilt, the unease. Eubank has been here before, as has his old coach, Ronnie Davies, who tonight happens to be sitting by the door, arms folded, angered to be going through it all again. He's one man in the hubbub who fails to see an upside to what transpired. 'His corner should have pulled him out of there or the referee should have stopped it,' Ronnie growls. 'That boy took way too much punishment.'

Eubank stops pacing the floor to nod his head in agreement.

'I thought he should have been stopped around the seventh,' Davies goes on. 'He was just getting beaten up. He was getting thrashed. It was a severe beating. I thought

Eubank was unbelievable, I thought he was great, but I don't feel happy right now.'

At the end of round eight, Eubank, the father, had teased a smile of contentment and then climbed into the ring, careful not to dirty his black designer suit. He was now standing in the corner, front and centre, just how he likes it. There was a light above him, a camera nearby. He knew it was on. He could feel the heat. He sensed the world watching. And yet, while usually his cue to act up, do something only Chris Eubank would do, become in equal parts pantomime dame and villain, he seemed less playful than normal, less aware of his stage, less keen to grab it. His expression was serious, perhaps one of concern – not for his son, he'd say, but for the opponent. When he spoke, even his trademark lisp straightened out; never had his enunciation been clearer. These were evidently words that needed to be heard and digested.

'If the referee doesn't stop it, I don't know what to tell you,' he said to Chris Junior in the corner. 'If he doesn't stop it, and you keep on beating him like this, one, he's getting hurt, and, two, if it goes to a decision, why hasn't the referee stopped the fight? I don't know why.' As the lecture continued, Ronnie Davies, Junior's official cornerman, applied Vaseline to the boxer's expressionless face. 'So maybe you shouldn't leave it to the referee. But you're not going to take him out to the face, you're going to take him out to the body. Okay?'

Satisfied, Eubank backtracked towards the centre of the ring, posed momentarily, and then used a handkerchief to wipe both his hands. As he did so, he studiously watched his son ready his mind for round nine.

'Seconds out.'

They all, at this point, have their preferred ending. Eubank, self-appointed director, scripts it so that his son will break up Nick Blackwell, the opponent, with body punches and bring about a respectable, PG-rated finish in the next round. He doesn't want to see Blackwell take further punishment, nor does he want to run the risk of his son being extended into the championship rounds unnecessarily. Everything should be just so. Clean, precise, his way.

His boy, however, has other ideas. Though the end result, a stoppage victory, is absolutely a shared goal, Junior, the maverick, wants to architect the finish on his terms. This means conclusively and painfully, certificate 18. He wants to make Blackwell pay for all he has said in the weeks preceding the fight; like all boxers, he wants a clean knockout, an addition to his highlight reel, but, better than that, he gets off on the idea of forcing Blackwell to quit, give up, do the very thing he swore he'd never do.

Across the ring, in Nick Blackwell's corner, the desired ending is somewhat more dramatic, not far off fanciful. This ending requires Nick, the underdog, successfully ignoring his broken nose and the fact he is partially sighted due to the grotesque haematoma above his left eye, and attacking Eubank Jr with a ferocity he has lacked all night, eventually wearing him down in the final rounds, engineering a stoppage and rendering the three judges' scorecards, all of which have Eubank Jr in front, redundant.

The referee, Scotland's Victor Loughlin, has his ending of choice, too. He, like most officials, prefers the idea of the judges taking responsibility, which is a way of saying he hopes the fight goes the distance, both men come away unscathed, and the rightful winner is the one who has landed the most punches. Loughlin, of course, will show no aversion to administering a stoppage, if need be, but so far neither man has been sufficiently troubled to warrant an intervention, and he would rather it stay that way until the final bell, for their sake, and for his.

As for the two and a half thousand people in the crowd, and the three million watching at home on Channel 5, their perfect ending is a combination of the above. The majority in the venue appear to want Blackwell to win, such is the polarising, aloof nature of the Eubanks, but they also fancy something dramatic. A decision win either way is acceptable, providing the action compensates for the lack of climax, but, deep down, regardless of the winner, there remains a hankering for the violent and the definitive. This is always the way.

What about the outcome *nobody* wants? In this instance, Eubank Jr continues to decorate Blackwell with shots, continues to rearrange his face, and then the referee, wincing at the state of the champion's left eye, asks the ringside doctor to inspect the damage in round ten. Seconds later, on the advice of the doctor, the fight is waved off. Boos ring out. Blackwell looks deflated. Even Eubank, the victor, experiences a momentary adrenalin dump. But soon it will get worse. The ending, that is. The *proper* ending. Soon it will go beyond just sport, winning and losing, and turn into a matter of life or death, as Nick Blackwell complains he feels dizzy and weak before collapsing to the canvas. This truly makes it the ending nobody wants. It's also the ending nobody saw coming.

Chris Eubank will argue this point. He'll claim he saw it coming from round seven, and that the call for his son to target Blackwell's body was a display of compassion motivated by such foresight. He may well be right. *But you're not going to take him out to the face, you're going to take him out to the body.* When unaware of the ending or, indeed, what happened to Chris Eubank in 1991, it's easy to consider this line nothing more than typical corner talk, the words of a man simply exploring the possibility of his boxer switching tactics mid-fight in an attempt to secure a finish. It is a call for creativity, a nudge towards Plan B, the matter-of-fact teachings of a trainer; Eubank, having been there himself, is telling his son he won't be able to take his opponent out with shots to the face – a path well travelled – and that he'd be better served trying something else. The mantra is clear.

When the narrative suddenly flips due to Blackwell's collapse, however, and Eubank loses control of it, so the context changes. *But you're not going to take him out to the face, you're going to take him out to the body.* Now the words can be interpreted differently. They can be perceived as the words of a father instructing his son to perform a certain action for the betterment of both himself and his opponent. Not a suggestion but a command. Less strategic, more emotionally led. *Do it or else! It's for your own good! And his!*

In a mark of the moment's weight, short video clips of this speech, originally shown on Channel 5, will go viral and divide the nation. The question that follows is a simple one: was Chris Eubank trying to save the life of Nick Blackwell? Hardened fight aficionados scoff at the very idea because they see the apparent method behind Eubank's monologue. Yet those unfamiliar with such trade vernacular come to believe Eubank's past – specifically, his near-tragic rematch with Michael Watson – has haunted a former champion to such an extent that he felt moved to not only protect Nick Blackwell but to also prevent his offspring from going through the same ordeal he experienced twenty-five years ago.

PROLOGUE

Motive irrelevant, the plan failed. Now, in the changing room after the fight, with his son still hidden from view, Eubank solemnly eats chunks of pineapple from a plastic container and circles the room. He occasionally glances over at Davies, his former coach, and though no words are exchanged the look alone says everything. In that moment, they think not just of Nick Blackwell but Michael Watson, the man whose life was changed irrevocably as a result of an uppercut Eubank landed on 21 September 1991 at White Hart Lane. It's the name on everyone's mind, in fact. The name nobody will dare say out loud.

'You can see I'm teary now, can't you?' Eubank says to me.

'You've been there,' I reply, figuring it's the safest way of welcoming Michael Watson into the conversation without mentioning his name.

Eubank wipes tears from his eyes and shakes his head. 'It's not that I've been there,' he says. 'I *am* there.'

During the course of this discussion, some thirteen and a half minutes after he left the ring on a stretcher, Nick Blackwell is placed in an induced coma. He then flatlines in the back of an ambulance.

THE BAD BOY

Before going any further I have a confession of my own to make. When, over a decade ago, I first expressed an interest in interviewing light-heavyweight boxer George Khalid Jones, it wasn't because he was coming off a loss to a former world champion, it wasn't because I'd briefly met him two years earlier when he was in England for sparring, and it wasn't even because I rated him all that highly as a perennial fringe contender. No doubt the southpaw from Paterson, New Jersey was a solid, dependable and dangerous veteran on his day, but his career alone certainly wasn't relevant or noteworthy enough to justify a two thousand-word, four-page feature in *Boxing Monthly* magazine circa spring 2006. Khalid probably knew that, too. He also knew that much of the reason why I, and presumably many others, had made contact with him of late had everything to do with the fact he killed a man in the ring in 2001.

Total infamy: he'd spent his entire boxing life wanting to be recognised, acknowledged and interviewed, just presumably not like *this*. Not on these terms. But, truth be told, his career was winding down, though it pained him to admit, and he knew there was every chance he'd bow out later that year best remembered for ending the life of Beethavean 'Bee' Scottland. There'd be no world title win to overshadow the incident and redefine him; he never even got the chance to fight for one. And there'd be no happy ending, either.

More often than not, then, calls made to George Khalid Jones would chew around the carcass of his 23–3–1 (wins–losses–draws) record before eventually getting to the last bit of meat: the tragedy. And what made Khalid's account all the juicier was that he himself was a reformed character, an ex-convict incarcerated for drug deals and attempted murders who was redeemed by boxing and then, in a cruel twist of fate, ended up with blood on his hands while doing the very thing that saved him. It was tragic. It made for a great story. Certainly, it was all the impetus I needed to track down his phone number and give him a ring one February evening.

In many ways, this particular interview was to become a microcosm of my relationship with the sport itself: on the one hand I am disturbed by my love affair with violence, not to mention my eagerness to live vicariously through fighters with beating hearts and loving families, yet, on the other hand, I am more than happy to see two men endure the necessary pain to qualify their match-up as a 'Fight of the Year' contender. A great fight, after all, often takes the concept of punishment to the extreme, but is somehow considered admissible – a job well done – if both disfigured warriors live to fight another day. It is then we convince ourselves this sport is not only normal but the greatest sport in the world.

Khalid's story was, to me, no different. It was alluring for all the wrong reasons. Death, drugs, guns, prison sentences, mean streets and broken homes. But these very things, like big punches slicing eyelids, breaking ribs or leading to concussions, were the cause of so much of my anticipation and excitement. I couldn't wait to hear of the horror, albeit from a safe distance.

Khalid, I learned, was no stranger to trouble. It shaped his life. He was born, as Khalid Kasib, into it. He was labelled it. He was raised in a troubled home in Paterson, New Jersey, a troubled area, to a drug-dealing father with twenty-six kids and a mother, Ruth Ann, who raised eight kids alone and took out life insurance on Khalid at the age of nine, so sure was she that he wouldn't make it much further (and they wouldn't be able to afford the inevitable funeral costs).

More trouble: Khalid, upon turning eleven, was forced out of his mother's house because it burnt down and then moved in with his father, who had abandoned him when Ruth Ann was six months pregnant. Shortly after this reshuffle, Khalid smoked his first marijuana joint with his father and was told, in no uncertain terms, that it was safer to do drugs this way because his father would always look out for him in the event of a bad trip. Knowing no better, Khalid thought it was cool, and so too did his friends, who often visited the house to score weed.

Khalid went deeper still from the age of thirteen. Now he was frequently playing poker face in taxis in order to ferry marijuana and cocaine to and from New York, again at his father's behest. Never was Khalid stopped during these missions. In fact, most of the time he'd complete the transactions with all the smoothness and composure of an old pro before returning to his father's house to enjoy the fruits of their labour. This meant sitting on the couch together, side-by-side, smoking crack cocaine. 'We called it "base shit" because you cook it up and base it with the chemicals,' he told me. 'At the time, you don't think you're addicted to the stuff, but, looking back now, I know I was.'

Thanks to his father, a shotgun was shoved down Khalid's throat at the age of fourteen and an addiction to heroin and crack soon consumed him. He was also reportedly on probation from the age of seven, but says, with no small amount of pride, that his first sentence in a youth correctional facility didn't arrive until the age of nineteen when he was locked up for shooting 'a guy who tried to rob me and a friend on a street corner'.

In total, at least as far as he can remember, Khalid was sent to jail for fourteen convictions of drug-taking and supplying, with the odd gun charge thrown in, and back and forth had over eleven years invested in the state penitentiary. By his own estimation, he was arrested eighteen or nineteen times, and called prison home from 1985 to 1989, 1990 to 1993 and 1997 to 2000.

One bright spot amid the darkness: Khalid eventually managed to undo some of his father's handiwork and wean himself off heroin. 'I haven't done heroin since the first of December 1991,' he said, proudly. His daughter, Aisha, was born a year and two months before that date and her mother left Khalid because he was doing twenty-one bags of heroin a day. He resented her for years, but now understands.

What's more, it was while in county jail, thus away from

his father, that Khalid finally started to find some direction and purpose in life. He first discovered that special food privileges, afforded only to boxers, included cheeseburgers and ice cream. He then discovered boxing. Fighting, of course, came naturally to him, it was something he'd been doing too much of on the streets, but to actually box – work behind an educated jab and explore the benefits of neat footwork – was an alien concept. He'd never spent time in an amateur boxing club, much less had a licensed fight.

Nevertheless, acting on the promise that the county jail boxing team had its own chef, Khalid started to shadowbox, lift weights and do press-ups on a regular basis, performing each with vigour, and then joined the team, beat all-comers and garnered a fearsome reputation within the prison. He ate well and was left alone.

It wasn't just fellow inmates and fighters on whom he left an impression. The boxing coach also liked what he saw. 'You don't have to keep fighting on the street,' he said to Khalid when he was about to leave the prison. 'You're good at it. Why do it for free?'

Khalid, at first, was suspicious. He didn't believe you could get paid for something he'd been doing on the streets since he was knee-high. It didn't add up. Nobody he knew made money from street-fights. But it was professional boxing he was being manoeuvred towards – prizefighting – and pretty soon Khalid was packed off to Minnesota for a paid fight against Marty Lindquist, an unbeaten local hope eager to feast on an ex-con with no amateur experience. It was September 1994 and Khalid was paid $400 for the gig. Not a king's ransom by any stretch, but still it blew his mind to think he was going to be fed crisp American dollar bills for something he'd have happily done for free. You know, a fist fight. One on one. What's known as your typical evening's entertainment in Paterson.

Four rounds later, Khalid had secured his first professional victory and silenced the Minnesota natives. The promoters were restless. They felt they'd been duped. 'They saw me as a bum with no amateur experience,' he said. 'I told them, "I had a hundred and fifty fights on the streets. Didn't they tell you that?"' All in all, the con with no name won his next ten pro fights, every one of them in the New Jersey area, before yet another three-year prison term sucker-punched him from out wide and disrupted his progress. He was off drugs, that was no longer the problem, but a replacement addiction had emerged in the form of gambling, which led to further bouts of drug-dealing and armed robbery; a need to pay debts owed to bookies saw Khalid juggle a promising boxing career with an equally unpromising life as a street hustler. Next thing he knew he was standing before a judge who told him, 'Mr Jones, you are a menace to society.'

Back in jail, back where he felt he belonged, Mr Jones soon encountered a Jewish counsellor by the name of Bobby Dickstein. It was now 1998 and, up to that point, Khalid had never stayed out of prison longer than two years and a third of his thirty-one years had been invested in jail. He was something of a regular. But Dickstein had heard all about him and wanted to help.

'A lot of the things he was saying sounded good to me, man,' Khalid said. 'I had a trust issue back then, but I gave it a chance and it worked. Since then I've never been back to prison, I've never broke the law, and he's helped me out with financial issues and showed me how to guide my money in the right direction. He was the first person who came into my life who wasn't around me because he needed something.

I always relied on people from the street. Street life was the norm. It was a lifestyle. I never thought a white guy would be the one to show me the way. But I also never knew anything about fatherhood, honesty or integrity before I met Bobby. He taught me things about fatherhood that my father never could have taught me. It took a white, Jewish guy to show me how to become a father to my kids and a husband to my wife.'

With the help of a white, Jewish guy, Khalid regained his momentum and thirst for fighting in 2000, when released from jail for the last time, having served thirty-four months of a four-year sentence, and won a further four fights to take his pro boxing record to 15–0. He was now, some believed, on the verge of an unlikely shot at the world light-heavyweight title. Hope, for once, was suddenly plentiful.

But then it happened. The fight. The reason for my phone call. The very thing that set Jones apart from other fighters with rough upbringings.

'Are you happy to talk about the Scotland fight?' I asked him in 2006.

'Sure,' he said. 'I *need* to talk about it.'

Such candour shocked me. 'Why is that?'

'Because going through that tragedy and meeting Bee's wife, Denise, changed my life for the better.'

Hold that thought.

After speaking to Khalid for an hour one Sunday evening in 2006, I was convinced of a few things. I was convinced that, at thirty-eight, he'd never box again. I was convinced he was a changed man (Khalid has, since 2003, benefitted from therapy sessions with Dr Stephen Garbarini, which have pulled him away from alcohol and patched up relationship issues). I was convinced his story was the greatest story in boxing. I was also convinced to start watching *The Wire*, at his request, in the hope I'd be able to better relate to life in the projects. Yeah, right. Finally, I was convinced I'd stay in touch with George Khalid Jones beyond our initial conversation, which I did (the best time to catch him is when he's driving one of the three trucks he owns on a long-distance voyage across New Jersey).

Above all that, though, Khalid made me realise death wasn't only a part of life, it was very much a part of boxing, too. It happens. All too often, some might say, but it happens. And it's tragic. And it's hard to talk about. And it raises countless questions. But it also changes people. Sometimes for the better, sometimes not. It changes those who witness it, those who fear it, and those who cause it. It changes certain aspects of the sport itself.

Death, one could argue, is as much a part of boxing's fabric as world titles, weight divisions, ten counts, three judges and twelve rounds, and to deny its existence is to do a disservice to the men and women who willingly fight to within an inch of it for our satisfaction and applause. Khalid taught me that in 2006. He killed a man in the ring and hated himself for it. But, as a professional fighter, he also knew he had a job to do and that it could so easily have been him taken too soon. For that reason, he had no issue discussing it.

Similarly, Khalid saw no issue with sending me a DVD copy of an interview he did with ESPN in which he spoke in detail about the Scotland incident and how it had impacted upon his life. The DVD arrived roughly a week after our chat and was received with enthusiasm and appreciation. Though I hardly knew the man, nor cared much about the ups and downs of his career, the greater subject matter, death, by now gripped me. It was taboo; boxing taken to its extreme; the thing the fight fraternity knew existed but refused to acknowledge unless it was completely necessary; the thing they didn't want you to see. So, feeling rebellious, I fished out the documentary's companion piece – a copy of the fight itself – and one night created my own Jones vs. Scottland double bill. Fight followed by documentary. I chose to do so not because I was writing a feature about Jones – that was already in the can – but simply because I was intrigued and had never before seen, on television or in person, a fight in which one of the two boxers sustained injuries so severe they would later perish. I was nineteen. Teenagers do strange, disturbing shit like that. It's why websites such as LiveLeak exist.

The done thing is to say it was horrible. *Really* horrible. The fight, a match between a fully fledged light-heavyweight and a natural super-middleweight, was one dominated by booming uppercuts thrown by Jones and swallowed by Scottland, and one which ended in dramatic fashion with thirty-seven seconds left to run. The accompanying documentary, meanwhile, serving to add context and a drop of humanity to the barbarism, made it seem all the more devastating, all the more real.

At least, that would have been the case had I not been nineteen years of age and so far removed, physically and emotionally, from the tragedy. Had I not been obsessed with the spectacle of two people fighting in a ring, the only set-up whereby one human being can legally kill another. Had I not been a fan of fights; regulated fights, unregulated fights, hockey fights, bullfights, catfights, playground fights, pub fights, pillow fights, food fights, all fights. I was, at this stage, untarnished, yet to be spooked by witnessing a death or even a serious injury in the ring, and this allowed me to disconnect and compartmentalise what I was watching on screen. There was a fight, a mismatch, some heavy punches, a knockout and then a bad, bad ending. But that, in the eyes of an ignorant and insensitive juvenile, was about the extent of it. A stranger died. It was sad. It could have been the other guy, the one dishing out the beating, but that night he had the smaller man's fortunes on his side. This is boxing. Let me see the knockout again, just to make sure.

Ten years later, on the cusp of turning thirty, this book represents my aversion therapy, my behaviour-modification treatment, the jolt to the system I probably require. To reference *A Clockwork Orange*, I am Alex and this book is Ludovico's Technique; meaning that as a consequence of meeting and interviewing boxers who have killed in the ring, and in some cases taking them back to the venue in which a tragedy occurred, I may well become conditioned to falling severely ill at the very thought of ultraviolence. 'It's quite simple really,' the nurse will say, 'we're just going to show you some films.'

While inherently sceptical, I want to discover if it works. I want to know if visiting traumatised boxers and haunted houses and watching footage of other ring tragedies will alter the way I view an extreme sport I have at times trivialised, taken for granted and consumed purely as escapism. I'm prepared. I'm subservient. I'm eager to be diagnosed and, if necessary, fixed.

In search of answers, I will be injected with a serum, stuffed in a straightjacket and strapped down like Hannibal Lecter. My eyelids will be then be prised open and pegged back to allow eye drops to hit my eyeballs from close range. This also prevents me looking away.

Images and tales of violence follow; a real horrorshow. Ludwig van Beethoven's Ninth Symphony plays.

The Start.

2

THE NOBLE ART
(OF ME HURTING YOU)

One... two... three... four... five... hands cupped around his mouth, he's counting jabs. Only jabs. Nobody has the faintest idea why. But as left hands snake out from the hip of his son, quickly, sneakily, as if picking a commuter's pocket, the father in the navy suit, white shirt, salmon bow-tie, skin-tight denim jeans and oversized black winklepickers, his cane temporarily set against a nearby table, tallies them up. In doing so, he sounds like a dance teacher counting steps. He sounds like a teacher, full stop. He also sounds unhinged. It's not even as though the jabs are landing. They're not. Some fall short, others deflect off the arms and gloves of the sparring partner. This is, therefore, no celebration of success. Six... seven... eight... nine... ten... the sparring partner, a reigning Commonwealth and former British super-middleweight champion, must by now, I figure, be somewhat distracted, if not downright irritated, by the lisping voice at ringside. Of all the possible narrators, he surely thinks. But father and son seemingly don't care how *he* feels. To them, this is imperative. It's part of the lesson. Eleven... twelve... thirteen... fourteen... fifteen... interestingly, even the son now seems tired of being observed, of being judged, of being counted. It shows in his stern, sullen face and in the way he all of a sudden limits the use of that particular punch, the jab, in favour of unleashing flashier hooks and crosses. Shots that, you know, aren't counted. Sixteen... seventeen... eighteen... nineteen... twenty... the buzzer sounds to signal the end of the first round *and* the counting. Chris Eubank grins in the direction of his son, Chris Junior, and waves his index finger in a manner which reveals he's satisfied. Twenty jabs, it seems, was the requisite amount.

In the corner, Ronnie Davies, the rosy-cheeked, shuffling and long-suffering trainer of two generations of Eubanks, wipes Junior's face with a towel and offers him a shot of water from a two-litre bottle. 'Suck it up,' he says. Junior frowns and walks away. There was likely a tut as well. Back turned, he spits, 'That doesn't even mean anything.' There's definitely a snarl, a look of general disdain, and Ronnie, a man in his sixties, remains perceptive enough to detect it. 'Tell him, Eubank!' he shouts to the father, a request greeted by two hands in the air, a shrug and a smile that indicates he, the father, is unsure how to tame the beast that roams before them.

The son doesn't seem to require help, advice, encouragement or throwaway clichés. He's four fights into a professional boxing career, already both helped and hamstrung by his famous fighting surname, and appears to know his path. Upon arriving in the gym, one situated beneath a railway arch in Vauxhall, he'll offer a cursory handshake and nothing more. Not a smile, not chit-chat, not a look of acknowledgement. He broods. He scowls. You are all his enemy. Sometimes he won't even bother with the handshake. This is work, not a social. You are not people with whom he would voluntarily choose to spend time, his dead eyes seem to say.

Even today, when surrounded by family – his father, his brother, Sebastian, and Ronnie, a man the Eubanks certainly consider 'family' – Chris Junior ploughs on alone, oblivious to them all. There are no attempts from anyone to distract Junior, converse with Junior or lighten Junior's mood. Instead, they give him a wide berth. Let Junior be Junior.

He stands before a mirror and flares his nostrils. He then checks his face for bumps, bruises and general blemishes, working on areas that displease him, and begins the ritual of wrapping his hands. Without any help, Junior covers his fists with wraps and then applies to his knuckles each of the strips of white tape he had earlier hung from the edge of the long wall mirror; an impressive sight to behold, not far off an art form, he has clearly practised this process on his own many times before. Cold. Insular. Driven. Unapologetic. They are all words his father will later use to describe him. And all ring true in this moment.

Back to the action. The counting stops and round two is all the better for it. George Groves, the paler-than-alabaster sparring partner, settles down and demonstrates a searching jab of his own. Taller, heavier and vastly more experienced, the Groves jab boasts a seasoning and sharpness Eubank Jr's lacks, and is used sparingly to control and dictate. It is a range-finder. It has purpose: quality, not quantity.

Eubank Jr, however, maintains perks of his own. Physically imposing and athletically blessed, he closes the distance on

Groves and rips him to the body and head with uppercuts and hooks, at times shoving him against the ropes and pinning him in corners. It's visceral, violent stuff. There's a ferocity to Eubank Jr's attacks normally absent in sparring sessions. In his mind, this is no practice. This is a fight.

The round ends and his father again struggles to contain his delight. He claps his hands and connects his thumb and index finger to flick an A-OK sign in the direction of Ronnie. 'Spot on, son,' he purrs. 'Spot on.'

Now it's Groves' turn to get belligerent. Dressed down by his trainer, Adam Booth, he aggressively bumps into Eubank Jr at the restart, perhaps to remind him who he is and where they are, and then continues this physicality for the next three minutes, dictating the action behind his jab and landing consecutive rights on Eubank Jr's face. Groves nods his head. He's satisfied. The unwilling recipient, meanwhile, opens his arms wide, as though sunbathing upright, and then beats his chest in a display of simultaneous pride and annoyance.

Watching on, his father becomes restless. A frown forms across his brow and he moves perilously close to creasing his designer suit against the dusty ring canvas. 'Nice, George,' he says, as Groves pivots out of a corner and crashes a counter right hand against the skull of his son. Booth is also heartened by what he sees. 'He's reacting to your movement, George!' he extols. 'That's a skill!'

Out for round four, Junior, detecting his father's sudden anxiety, bites down, works harder and punches in combination with renewed vitality. He sets about Groves, chases him, smothers him. Groves, in contrast, perhaps drunk on his earlier success, gets careless, allows himself to be clipped with a long and explosive left hook, and then

14

grinds to an immediate halt. Embarrassed, not hurt, he shakes his head, drops his hands and allows Eubank Jr the luxury of landing a further flurry of shots on his unguarded head, snapping it this way and that; an act of bravado, for he wants to show his toughness, it is also motivated in large part by frustration.

Clearly, Chris Eubank hates what he sees. He waves his hands in the air and tries to catch George's attention. 'No, no, no!' he shrieks. 'George, what are you doing?! Why give a man a free shot like that?!' The two boxers, of course, carry on sparring. They continue taking turns to hit one another around the head and body. They are numb to external forces, lost in battle. But the former world champion at ringside, the man who once meticulously counted jabs for an entire round, has now lost all interest. His mind wanders. So do his feet. 'You don't give up free shots in this sport, George!' he yells for a second time, marching around the ring. 'Protect yourself at all times!'

He waits for the round to end before moving close to Groves and Booth by the corner. 'See that bravado?' he says, enraged.

There's no answer back from the fighter. Not even so much as acknowledgement of his presence. He views Eubank only as a nuisance at this time.

'Would you do that in a fight, George?'

Again there is no reply.

'No, you wouldn't! So why do it now? Don't give anyone a free shot. *Ever*!'

The irony of Chris Eubank of all people, once showman extraordinaire, imploring a young fighter to remain orthodox and protected at all times was not lost on the two men enduring the wrath of an ex-champion, nor was it lost on me. It was perhaps why Groves and Booth refrained from answering.

Far tougher to ignore his presence, though. He was so vehement, so infuriated, so emotional. Understandable, you might say, if it had been his son getting macho and acting up. *Then* he'd have every right to show distress and tell him off. But this wasn't like that. This was entirely different. Indeed, his son *had* done something similar only the round before. He too had dropped his hands when caught by a punch. Yet, in that instance, his father remained calm and trusted his son to fix his error. There was only ever a look. Why, then, the sudden concern for the more experienced opposite number? Was it ego? Was it a need for control? Did he want to exert his power and expertise? Or did Chris Eubank genuinely care about the well-being of the person with whom his son was trading blows?

All questions were left unanswered when I departed Vauxhall back in the summer of 2012. They were questions I dared not ask of people I hardly knew. But, regrettably, four years later, while in the midst of writing about ring tragedies and their repercussions, having never experienced one myself, I'd begin to understand.

Only three punches were necessary. One broke the man's eye socket, the other broke his jaw and the third broke his nose. Like that, the damage was done. Nick Blackwell, then seventeen, required no further invitation to hunt his wounded prey and knock him out.

Round one, fight over, he looked down at the man; a nutcase, a thug, two stone heavier than he was, many years older, bald, tattooed, the archetypal opponent encountered on the unlicensed circuit. Blackwell, the victor, smiled, proud to have prevailed in a so-called mismatch he was expected to lose, and recalled how beforehand, before the cracked jaw, the busted eye socket and the crooked nose, before the bloodshed, those at ringside had felt sorry for him. One concerned spectator even cried, 'What are you doing? He's only seventeen!'

Eight years later, Blackwell, the reigning British middle-weight champion, decides to spar topless. He decides to spar topless because he is immensely proud of his current physique – fit, healthy, toned to perfection, no sign of a pinchable inch – and because he wants to prepare his abdomen, his ribs, his liver, his kidneys, his chest and his arms for war. He wants to feel the punches of sparring partner George Groves and for them, the hurtful blows, to toughen his skin and his resolve. He also wants to go back in time, back to when he was seventeen and bloodthirsty, back to when he was beating up grown men in unlicensed scraps. 'My first-ever fight was a bloodbath, like a bare-knuckle fight with gloves,' he reminisces, a glint in his eye. 'Those watching couldn't believe how bloody and brutal it was.'

The ten rounds Blackwell and Groves share in Hammersmith bring to mind the rounds I used to watch Eubank Jr and Groves serve up in Vauxhall all those years ago. They are fast-paced and frenetic. There are innumerable momentum shifts. Neither man appears to get the upper hand for any longer than a few seconds. Give and take, back and forth, at times it's hard to watch; you remind yourself it's only sparring, not a fight, and you take comfort in that; you fear for the pair of them if their gloves were downsized from sixteen-ounce sparring gloves to ten-ounce fight-night gloves and, of course, if their head-guards were removed.

DOG ROUNDS

Here's the subtext, though, the secret kept from all in the gym: irrespective of the head-guard and bigger gloves, Nick Blackwell, in taking repeat prescriptions of heavy punches, is soon concussed. It's the reason why he's going to suddenly feel sluggish and the reason why he'll sleep in the car on the way home. It's the reason why the next day he'll forget he even sparred Groves. It's the reason why he will experience dizziness and light-headedness and fall ill. It's the reason why he shouldn't fight in ten days.

'I feel tired today,' he says in his West Country accent as he dries his face and body with a towel and rests on the leather sofa in Groves' plush gymnasium. 'It took three hours to get here and I didn't want to get out the car.'

Nick travelled from Cardiff with his close friend Jake, but was forced to leave behind his coach, Gary Lockett, due to the Welshman contracting a common cold which had swept the gym, a cold Nick feared picking up so close to the fight (it would render him bed-bound two days later, in fact).

'He's got a lovely jab,' Blackwell says of Groves. 'When you get hit with one of those, it's like being hit by a right hand. So powerful and sharp. He's clever, too. He can control you inside quite well.'

'George has been boxing a long time,' I say. 'Unlike you, he has been boxing since he was a kid. He had a lot of amateur fights.'

'Yeah, that's true. I'm still learning.'

His comrade, Jake, sits beside him and tells me about the time the troublemaking Trowbridge Two went to Marbella, Spain to train alongside an established camp of boxers – champions, contenders, veterans – only to realise experience isn't everything. 'Oh, that lot were so patronising to begin with,' he says. 'They saw us as a couple of country bumpkins who trained themselves and didn't know what they were doing. They asked, "Are you sure you want to join us on this run?" They made it out to be some big deal. What happened, Nick?'

'We smashed 'em,' says Nick. 'It was easy.'

'Nick was finished by the time they were at the halfway point. It was embarrassing. I wasn't far behind and I'm no professional athlete. That's when we knew Nick was doing all right and was fitter than every fucker out there.'

On cue, Blackwell, full of life, watches Groves and his trainer, Shane McGuigan, son of Barry, prepare an abs session and miraculously comes alive again. 'I'll have some of that!' he exclaims. The champion professedly can't get enough of it, enough of this – the training, the sparring, the grind. Though his body seems as fit and as healthy as it can be, and even carries a kind of golden shine, he's still a number of pounds over the middleweight limit and aware of the need to keep working, keep pushing, keep sweating. It's not yet time to stop. There are still ten days to go.

Nick Blackwell's life has been like this since he first entered The Ringside Gym (now The Contender Gym) in Trowbridge at the age of fifteen. He went with his younger brother Dan, and fell apart in his first sparring session. Fifty-four seconds into it, he estimates. But, whatever the actual length of time Blackwell was able to keep his arms pumping, there was a determination to his character that endeared him to his coach, Mark Kent, and it wasn't long before he was given the green light to start competing.

No ordinary competition, Blackwell was about to embark on a brief but brutal white-collar career and amass eighteen fights in total. He was oblivious to the concept of amateur boxing, kept away from head-guards, and was instead led to the slaughter in ten-ounce gloves for £150 a pop. Every one of his opponents would be older than him, bigger than him, heavier than him, but Blackwell, at seventeen, could see no better way of making money. He was making money *and* beating people up. It was win–win, certainly preferable to the college course he was taking with a view to become a bricklayer.

Unknowingly, Nick's unlicensed debut would consist of not one but two fights. The first was against a man half a stone heavier than him, yet this counted for little as he was knocked out inside a round, and the second also involved a heavier opponent, an army lad, one covered in tattoos, who was again dispatched soon after the fight had begun. Blackwell took to fighting with unnerving ease. He seemed made for it. He wanted more. At eighteen, he turned professional.

When he returns to the sofa, having completed his abs workout, Nick is tired but talkative. It always seems to be the way with him. Personable almost to a fault, he makes time for everyone, calls them all either 'mate' or 'matey', and can have even a stranger feeling as if they will soon become the closest of friends. Maybe it's the loneliness of the prizefighter.

'I just feel like I have no social life whatsoever at the moment,' he says, shaking his head. 'This thing – boxing – takes up all your time. I haven't had a proper holiday for ten years.'

He's nearly seven years into his professional career and has won nineteen of twenty-three fights.

'Seriously,' he adds, 'I don't do anything but go to the gym, eat and sleep. I've got no time for people. No time for family, friends, anything. You do start thinking, "Will my life always be like this?" It's a bit of a worry.'

'You've only got to do it for a few more years,' I say. 'You can have a social life in your thirties.'

'We want him out in a couple of years, don't we?' says Jake.

'That's the thing,' says Nick, 'you feel happy to sacrifice stuff when you're a kid. But I'm twenty-five now. I feel like I'm running out of time. It won't be long before I'm thirty.'

'Still five years,' I say.

'It only feels like yesterday I was twenty.'

'Are you looking after your money?'

'Yeah, much better than I used to. After losing to Martin Murray in 2011, I got really depressed. I got paid £12,500 and it was my biggest payday, but I spent it all very quickly and was then on a massive downer. I didn't think I was good enough to be a boxer. I thought I'd have to get a normal job.'

'And now?'

'I want to start looking for a house or a flat or an apartment after this fight. I want to move to Cornwall.'

'Why Cornwall?' I ask, aware of his newfound love of surfing.

'I've always been a water baby,' he says. 'When it's sunny, I feel like I need to hit the beach and I love being in Cornwall. It's relaxed, it's chilled and you can just get away from everyone. I'm not a city boy. I like to be in the country.'

He plans to go surfing in Cornwall immediately after his next fight, believing it will offer his body the chance to wind down and his mind the chance to distance itself from thoughts pertaining to combat. One extreme to the other. 'When you're down in Cornwall, you start turning soft,' he explains. 'You don't need that if you're a boxer. You've got to be hard. But I think that's why I like surfing. It takes you away from boxing completely. I feel at home down there, like that's where I should be. But, then again, when I'm training hard and getting my head punched in, I feel like that's also where I should be.'

This is clear just watching him fight, for never has a fighter appeared to truly *enjoy* the experience of giving and receiving punishment in the ring as much as 'Bang Bang' Blackwell. His smile is constant. It's present when he's winning; it's present when he's losing. For him, the ability to fight and make a living from doing so is the *real* victory. I mean, it wasn't that long ago he was falling short in British and Commonwealth title fights, desperately taking any short-notice opportunity that came his way, and generally slipping down snakes as opposed to climbing ladders. Reputation built more on successful sparring sessions than fight-night brilliance, Blackwell seemed destined to forever have to do things the hard way. He'd rack up countless rounds sparring the likes of Carl Froch and James DeGale, world super-middleweight champions, but then exhibit his own work in low-key fights from the insecurity of the away corner. He was both a paid sparring partner and paid opponent. Very little was ever on his terms.

In 2015, however, this started to change. He signed with promoter Mick Hennessy, which ensured him a terrestrial television platform on Channel 5, and then he won the British middleweight title with a shock seventh-round stoppage of highly touted Londoner John Ryder at the O2 Arena. He came from behind to score the upset. He dug in. He persevered. The performance, to some degree, encapsulated his entire career. And, from there, it only got better. Now a headliner in his own right, Blackwell knocked out another unbeaten fighter, Damon Jones, in the sixth round of a title defence in Derby, and then outlasted Jack Arnfield in a twelve-round brawl in Bristol. And *still* British middleweight champion. It had a ring to it.

Nick's arrival at Hennessy Sports coincided with my own, as press officer rather than boxer, and I was consequently now in the privileged position to work on each of his British title fights. More than that, I got to know Nick as a person. He became a friend within the sport. We communicated on a semi-regular basis, even if most of the time I'd be hassling him for quotes or directing interview requests his way, and never once did he let me down or mess me about. 'No problem, matey,' he'd say time and time again. I remember wishing all boxers were like him.

For being so dependable and accommodating, he deserved better. His story was one I tried to push to newspaper editors and television producers on countless occasions but each time his face didn't seem to fit. Not yet, anyway. He wasn't from the right part of the country. He had a funny accent. He was *only* a British champion. He had defeats on his record. I heard it all. When that failed, watch him fight, I'd say. He's a throwback television fighter. Old-school. Imagine 'Boom Boom' Mancini with a West Country accent. Looks like a surfer, fights like a savage. But the sales pitch never really got us anywhere. Still he struggled to sell tickets. Still there were empty seats at his fights.

Realists, the two of us would sometimes console each other by going over the process: win the British title, defend it as headliner, defeat Chris Eubank Jr – his number one contender, the *name* in the division – and then prepare for the accolades, the pound notes and the stardom. Nick wasn't stupid. He knew victory over Eubank Jr, live on terrestrial television, would make him rich and famous. It simply had to. So that was the aim: date 26 March 2016, venue Wembley Arena.

'Right, matey, we're off,' he says, rising from the sofa and hoisting his sports bag over his shoulder. 'Three hours back, and that's if we don't hit any traffic.'

We say our goodbyes and I watch as Nick and Jake, still smiling, still ribbing each other and making light of *everything*, skip out of the gym and close the door behind them.

'Tough guy,' says Groves approaching from a distance. 'He's very fit and stays on you. It will be interesting to see how Eubank reacts to that pressure. He'll cope early, but I wonder what he'll be like late in the fight if he's not getting his own way.'

McGuigan, his coach, follows just behind. 'You controlled him quite well today, though, I thought.'

'Yeah, I felt good today.'

'You hit him with some big shots.'

'Yeah.'

'I worry for Nick in later years. He takes too many.'

For now all eyes are on him. The son. The next generation. It won't stay this way, of course, it rarely does, but he has this moment temporarily. He's centre stage, middle of the ring, shadowboxing, grunting and growling with each punch he throws, title challenge on the horizon, and the Dictaphone of a local reporter edges closer and closer to his face. It was his choice to do it like this, to be interviewed while warming up, and he's determined to make it work.

'Ronnie, stop talking!' Chris Eubank Jr shouts in the direction of his trainer, sat ringside at Hove Amateur Boxing Club. A call for quiet, it's also a sign of who's running the show, at least for now. At least until his father shows up in approximately five minutes.

THE NOBLE ART (OF ME HURTING YOU)

Eubank Jr himself was late. He kept Mike Legg from the *Argus* newspaper waiting for some half an hour in the other gym. 'He's always late,' went the theory. Even so, by the time Junior bundled through the door, got a feel for the gym, realised it wasn't warm enough for his needs and moved to a different and smaller one next door, there was evident relief on the face of the journalist. He was grateful his journey, albeit a short one, hadn't been in vain.

'What do you think of the beard?' Junior asks the reporter.

'It's different,' says Legg.

'Yeah, I'm normally clean-shaven.'

It's as close as they get to small talk. Quickly, Junior returns to his shell. He pops out left and right punches. He's keen to get down to work. Keener still to be left alone.

The gilet jacket on top of his black tracksuit indicates he's having a hard time shifting weight, as any boxer does a few days from fight night, and Junior impatiently awaits the first sign of sweat forming on his brow. It will tell him the place is warming up, and will vindicate his decision to switch from one gym to another.

Meanwhile, his sister, Emily, is next to enter the gym. She's not here to box, nor is she here to lose weight. Conversely, she seems hell-bent on testing her brother on a day he resents being tested. 'What are you doing?' he says as he clocks the packet of crisps and fizzy drink in his sister's hands. 'I don't want to be seeing you walking in here with that when I'm cutting weight!'

It's said with a smile, I think. There's at least some sense that he's only *half* serious. His sister, though, continues regardless. Crisps, open. Can, open. Junior can only shake his head and resume punching. 'It's not nice training on an empty stomach,' he says to nobody in particular.

Maybe he's consulting the heroes on the wall. Hardly starved of inspiration, there is, for starters, a mural of his father stood alongside Nigel Benn, and then there is one of 'Sugar' Ray Leonard, accompanied by the quote, 'Boxing is the ultimate challenge. There is nothing that can compare to testing yourself the way you do every time you step in the ring.' There are also pictures of Mike Tyson and Lennox Lewis and Evander Holyfield and just about every other iconic fight figure of the last forty years. *They* know how he feels. *They* can relate.

Suddenly, at around 2:45p.m., another walks through the door. This one hasn't been painted. He doesn't come equipped with a motivational quote (though is more than happy to supply one if requested). In actual fact, he's the boy's father, Chris Eubank Sr. The unique, unmistakeable, ubiquitous Chris Eubank Sr.

There are no words spoken. Not to his son or to anyone else in the gym. He, better than anyone, knows when it's time to be quiet. This is gym time. Business time. He's content, therefore, to watch his son stretch, shadowbox and casually move around the ring.

Junior, I'm sure, has spotted his presence. How can he not have? Senior's lime and charcoal tracksuit is a dead giveaway. It's a curious thing, too, that tracksuit. One part North Face jacket, one part Real Madrid Adidas bottoms, Eubank somehow makes them match; were it not for the different logos, you'd swear they came as one. The colours align. It's seamless.

Seamless is also the most appropriate way of describing the motion of Eubank hurrying from the back of the gym to the side of the ring upon realising his son is about to be interviewed. He's there in a flash. And it's only when I look to my right and see one of Junior's friends filming the interview on his phone that it starts to all make sense. The father is merely positioning himself in shot. He perches by the ring ropes, ensures the camera picks up his best side, and then contemplatively cups his chin in his right hand. After that, the interview begins. Junior speaks.

'If you don't take a risk, you'll never achieve anything,' he says, to which Senior nods. He likes the answer. It moves him to put a foot on the canvas and get even closer. One more step and he'll be through the ropes.

'What about the weight?' asks Legg, Dictaphone out in front. 'You mentioned you still need to lose some pounds...'

'This is boxing,' goes the reply. 'It's never easy. It's always a struggle.'

His father approves.

'It's never nice waking up and knowing you're not going to get satisfactory meals throughout the day and still have to train like a demon. I want my Krispy Kreme doughnuts.'

His father now stands directly beside the reporter. The hope is to grab his son's attention. He wants to get some sort of message across. Junior, oblivious, finds a rope and skips.

'Nick Blackwell has done some sparring with George Groves ahead of this fight,' says Legg. 'Have you also had top sparring in this camp?'

'I've had adequate sparring,' Junior says. 'Top sparring? No.'

'What sort of game plan do you have for a fighter like Blackwell?'

'You go into a fight with a game plan, get punched on the nose and it all changes. You have to be adaptable.'

Senior shakes his leg out as if preparing to train or fight.

He limbers up. Then he raises a hand to the ceiling, an instruction of sorts, and again tries to catch his son's eye.

'Do you feel you're being painted out to be the bad guy in this fight?' asks Legg.

'I'm not a bad guy. I'm a good guy. I'm just being me.'

His father smiles and crosses his arms.

'I'm going to represent England and fly the flag,' Junior continues. 'Blackwell ain't doing that. He walks down the street and no one knows him. I'm a patriot. Winning the British title will be a proud moment for me. I'm driven. I'm focused on achieving this goal. I have one friend, one girlfriend, and her name is boxing.'

There it is – the clincher, the conversion of the buzzer-beating clutch shot. Senior pumps his fist in the air in celebration. It's the greatest thing he has ever heard.

'I haven't heard that from him before,' he later tells me. 'If that's not your answer, you're flawed. You have to be obsessed with this. The guys who are focused, they don't beat us. The guys who are *really* focused, they don't beat us. Why? It's because we're obsessed.'

I follow him through to the other gym – larger, colder – and we end up in its office. Eubank takes a seat behind the desk, as if running the place, and instructs me to close the door behind us. Once settled, he waves his hand for me to commence the interrogation. It's almost controlling. But I don't mind. His head tilts back. Forget words, I can nearly see his thoughts through his nostrils. I question how and why the attention has so quickly turned from son to father. This wasn't my plan. Feature in mind for *The Ring* magazine, I was only supposed to see the son and speak to the son. You know, the one with a fight coming up. But here I am. I've deviated. He has got me. I'm on the end of a string.

'The most powerful way to describe how boxing is to me is to think of yourself as a fundamental Christian or someone who is deeply religious,' Eubank begins. 'That's how I position myself within the gymnasium. The gymnasium, for me, was like my church. I was devout. I went there and I worshipped. I didn't socialise. I didn't talk to people who went there. I didn't want to hear anything but leather on flesh. The art, the life. I wanted to get to the pearly gates and I got there. Because I was devout. Because I was obsessed.'

'Junior seems to have that same obsession,' I suggest. 'Is that fair to say?'

'I didn't detect it from an early age, but, in retrospect, like father, like son. That's the way I see it. The best way to learn is the hard way. If I give you only support, it will buckle you. Support networks are counterproductive in boxing. If you stand on your own two feet and you're not leaning, then you have a chance. I remember Mike McCallum saying to me, "He's a bad boy." A bad boy means he's got energy, he's special. It means someone you don't mess with.'

But was his son truly standing on his own two feet if his father was within earshot of *everything* he said? I ask him if he ever worries he might be *too* supportive.

'Too supportive?' he says, refusing to entertain such a concept. 'How can I be *too* supportive? I am his father. He is me. You become your father as you get older. We're trying to be extraordinary.'

'What's your son like to be around? Is there a danger he can become too insular, too obsessed?'

'No, no, no,' says Eubank. 'He's happy-go-lucky. He's militant but he's easy to be around. You can get on with him fine, just don't bring up boxing. If you bring up boxing, the shutters come down. He's cold. Insular. Driven. Warmonger.

And unapologetic. He believes in the universal law which goes like this: for every action, there is an opposite and equal reaction. Don't mess with me and I won't mess with you. That's Junior. I'm a bit different. If you mess with me, I'll try and win you over. I'm going to make you a better man. I'll say, "Listen, don't do that. You hurt me, man." Whatever they say about me, it's not true. I'm just a guy. I want to get on with people. It's better that we're friends. Junior doesn't have that spirit.'

'Has Junior ever told you to ease off?'

The father frowns. It's another idea he can't comprehend. 'I'll leave you with this,' he says. 'I want you to find the clip of me speaking to Gary Newbon after the first [Nigel Benn] fight. My bottom lip quivers and I've done it. I've told my father I love him. I've said to my brother he said I couldn't do it, but I've done it...' Eubank nods proudly, then raises a finger. 'I want you to look at the people in the picture...' He pauses again. His eyes well up and his voice starts to crack. 'Where was *my* daddy? Where were *my* brothers? Where were *my* childhood friends? I had no one around.'

I see.

'I'll *never* do that to my boy. I don't want him to ever say, "Dad, where were you? Was there someone more qualified than you, Dad?" My dad's gone. He died in 2000. It took me years to realise that when I won that world championship he must have been a man of five foot three walking ten foot tall. He wouldn't have been able to buy a drink in Peckham or Brixton. "Eubank, the champion, that's the man's son," they'd say. He should have been in my pictures. So when they say I'm stealing my son's limelight, you're *goddamn right*.'

Back at Hove Amateur Boxing Club a decade ago, the

fifteen-year-old son of Chris Eubank wasn't quite sure why he was paired with a sparring partner four years older than him, with some twenty amateur bouts to his name, but now suspects it had everything to do with the fact he was the fifteen-year-old son of Chris Eubank. Certain assumptions were, of course, made because of this. They assumed the kid could fight. They assumed he was tough like his old man. They assumed he could take a beating.

But it never quite worked out like that. Instead, Chris Junior was 'absolutely battered' for three rounds, as if some point was proven in the process, and then exited Hove Amateur Boxing Club dismantled, dispirited and in disarray.

Or so they thought.

The teenager had other ideas. He made a pact with himself that it would never happen again and that he'd return to the gym at the next available opportunity and continue going there until *he* was the one dishing out the beat-downs. It was a promise he kept, too. Using the humbling as a catalyst, Eubank Jr stuck around, surrendered to his competitive spirit and quickly made the necessary improvements. He learnt how to box.

Fighting had never been a problem for Junior. It was in his DNA. It came naturally. But, that said, a propensity to gravitate towards unlicensed punch-ups isn't necessarily a positive thing and one street fight, in particular, was uploaded to YouTube in 2007, attracted over 130,000 views, and let the world know Chris Eubank's boy was mixed up with the wrong crowd.

'I knew I needed to escape those people and those situations as I was being led towards a dark place and boxing was the only thing that could save me,' he says. 'While I knew how to fight, I was now learning to box. It's different. I had to learn how to control my temper in the ring and fight without emotion.'

Although the child of a world champion prizefighter, Junior was shielded from the sport that defined his father. He didn't watch any of his fights. He didn't watch boxing, full stop. It was a dirty secret, something his father kept locked in a safe away from prying, inquisitive eyes. It was, he thought, for the best. Besides, Junior didn't exactly fight for the right. Even when he started boxing at fifteen there was no sudden urge to actually sit down and watch the sport on tape. He just didn't seem that way inclined.

'At first my father was reluctant to allow me to attend training sessions,' Junior recalls. 'He didn't understand why I was doing it and, of course, he knew just how hard the sport was. He didn't want me to experience the same sacrifice and hardship he went through. As time went on, though, he began to see how seriously I was taking it and how much I was improving, and that was when he started to warm to the idea. He needed to know I wasn't just mucking around and that I had some potential. Obviously, when he said he didn't want me to box, it only made me want to box even more. Like any young kid, I wanted to know more about this thing he told me to stay away from. I wanted to see if it was as extreme as he said it was.'

In order to seal the deal, the father tested his son's resolve, first by denying him the opportunity, and then, when issuing the green light, packing him off to America at just seventeen years of age to learn from the best in the business. A daunting prospect for most teenagers, Junior embraced the move with brio and appreciation. And, uncharacteristically, a smile. 'The time I spent in Vegas, training and living, is what has made me the fighter I am today,' he says.

In total, along with younger brother Sebastian, he spent four years stateside. Their father's acquaintance, Ms Irene Hutton, became their court-appointed legal guardian, they attended Spring Valley High School and they travelled the Vegas gyms working with some of the best trainers and fighters in the world; two years with three-weight world champion Mike McCallum was followed by a stint with Floyd Mayweather Sr, meaning Junior, on a daily basis, shared boxing rings with world champions such as Zab Judah, Chad Dawson and Montell Griffin. He'd take his ass-whuppings, his licks, his lessons, and he'd come back for more. School was in session. He loved every minute of it. He left a boy and returned a man. Better still, he returned a fighter.

'My dad knew it would be good for me to go to the States as an unknown, with no pressure, in order to learn my trade away from the spotlight,' he says. Oddly enough, Chris Senior, a street-fighter and occasional shoplifter raised by his father in south London, had been sent to live with his mother in the South Bronx, New York at a similar age. 'I was able to keep my head down out there and, although I was in Vegas, there were very few distractions,' Junior continues. 'But I wasn't with my family or friends and that is always tough. I just kept thinking that if I was able to survive that experience and come out the other side a better boxer and man, it would have been worthwhile. In boxing terms, I knew I'd be on another level to other young prospects when I returned to England.'

While stateside, Junior effectively replicated his father, a 1984 New York Golden Gloves champion, by winning the Nevada State Golden Gloves title in just his sixth amateur fight and the Western States Golden Gloves in his eighth. Then, once back home, he bagged the International

Haringey Cup in June 2011 and concluded his brief but fruitful amateur career with a record of 24–2. Both defeats were avenged.

The promising amateur turned professional as the twenty-two-year-old son of Chris Eubank in November 2011. What's more, in choosing Tina Turner's 'Simply the Best', effectively his father's theme tune, as his ring-walk music, and in choosing to vault the top ring rope, a move again made famous by his father, there was an unapologetic sense of the torch being passed.

'I've been jumping the ring ropes like that since day one,' Junior argues when pressed on this matter. 'I did that for my first amateur fight and have been doing it ever since. Nobody told me to do it. It's just something I've always done. The song choice was a group decision, though. At first I wasn't too sure about it, to be honest, but we talked it through and collectively felt the fans would appreciate it. In the end, I think it worked. It was a nostalgic ring entrance and the presence of my father obviously helped a lot, too. When my dad stood in front of the camera and then moved away to reveal me, it was telling people that he was then and this is now.'

Discussing similarities between himself and his father would, one assume, rank high on the list of Junior's least favourite things. Whenever pushed that way, his answers on the subject are delivered with a sigh and a roll of the eyes and are often monosyllabic. Perhaps such questions are too obvious and lazy. Or perhaps they simply act as a reminder that no matter how successful he is in his own career, he will never be able to swerve idle comparisons. He will never be able to fully escape the shadow.

'Of course, there will be similarities,' he says. 'I am his

son and we share the same blood and DNA. Things might not be exactly the same, but if you watch the way I punch and move, I'm sure you will pick up similarities. It's just a natural thing. His movement and ring generalship was truly impressive, and that is something I have definitely taken from him.'

Eubank Jr is now twenty-six and all grown up. He has since won twenty-one of twenty-two pro fights, the one blemish a points loss to Billy Joe Saunders in 2014, and is out to claim one of the few belts that eluded his father during his career – the British title. Look past the vaulting of the top rope, the fleeting fondness for Tina Turner, and the mid-fight posturing, and he is unquestionably his own man. Or at least should be by now. Little does he know, however, the father–son comparisons will soon only grow stronger.

His dad and I resume our chat the next day, this time not in Brighton but in Wembley, where we meet moments after his son's latest pre-fight press conference has concluded. I ask for another five minutes and Eubank, having traded the tracksuit for a blazer and jeans, gives me slightly more than that. I guilt-trip him into it, I suppose, by telling him the majority of the quotes he'd given me the day before, when holed up inside a gym's office, had then been rehashed, almost verbatim, while he was sat at the top table addressing the nation's media. He tries to argue the point – clarifying they were pearls of wisdom *everyone* needed to hear – but I'm not having any of it. I need more gold, I say.

Ego sufficiently massaged, he gives in. We leave the room and find a quiet corridor.

'Are you ever worried for Junior's health in this game?' I ask.

'I am not worried about Junior in this regard because

he is the danger,' replies Eubank, leaving just enough of a pause for the thought to register. 'Watch what I say. Junior is a *very* dangerous man. In this four-cornered circle where the objective is to score points by hitting your man, he's a very dangerous young man. And he wants to be dangerous. He is building himself to be dangerous. I talk to him about speed and tell him speed is power, but he wants power. He's working towards it. I mean what I say. Starting from this interview here now, watch what happens on Saturday.'

It almost seems a threat. Is he pre-empting a boxing match or a school shooting? *We Need To Talk About Junior*. He isn't smiling. He is serious. A chill runs down my spine.

'Were you the same kind of animal?'

'Definitely not,' he says. 'I *looked* fierce. I was a great actor. How good? Great. My acting was superb. I could take the punches and I could deliver the punches. And I could stay in there and take a beating. I was actually real. But I wasn't mean-spirited. If I had someone in trouble, I'd back up. Junior has mean intentions, though. Bad intentions. He is real and he has that intensity and he is cold.'

'If Junior wasn't real and intense and cold, would you stop him from boxing?'

'If you don't have the right attitude for the job, if you're ill-equipped, don't be in here. It's too dangerous. There have been many tragedies. There have been many deaths. It's a very dangerous business. Do you think I want my son entering boxing thinking he can take and not be taken? You *can* be taken. I'd rather you were mean-spirited to your core. I want him to take them before they take him. I want him to have that attitude.'

'It's a ruthless business,' I say.

'Yes, but there's a kindness in beating a man badly. That

kindness is based on correctness. When I'm hitting you with shots, it's not really you, it's the art of me hurting you. The art of me breaking you. It's the art of me pulling the spirit out of you. There's kindness in that, there's truth in that. That's deep. It's profound. But it's true. There is a kindness in letting a man "go". He would do it to you. It's a very dangerous game, a very dangerous business. If you have the ability to be so far above, in terms of ability, that you can hurt a man to his core but you don't, that shows how good you are at what you do and how thoughtful you are in the process. People think it's two men hitting each other. Far from it.'

His index finger, held directly in front of my face, declares he's not quite done yet. He takes a deep breath. His eyes close momentarily, only to then reopen. 'One of the most powerful lessons I was ever given happened in 1983. I was about seventeen years old, had just beaten someone, and I said to my mother, "Mum, I won the fight." The words she said became a part of me. They formed my mindset. She said to me, "What happened to the other boy?" I said, "Mum, why are you talking about him? I won!" She said, "*He* has a mother, too."'

THE
CROWDPLEASER I

Hamilton 'Rocky' Kelly walks alongside Matilda, his daughter, through the hotel lobby and towards a large conference room in which he used to fight. It's hard to know who's leading who. Matilda is ten, Rocky is fifty-two. She sips from a plastic bottle of Coca-Cola and seems completely disinterested in the matter at hand, whereas Rocky, dressed smartly for his big day in jeans and a collared shirt enhanced by specks of bright green and pink, carries a look of child-like wonder on his daughter's behalf.

His will forever be a fighter's face. The squashed flat nose; the taut, leathery brown skin; the scar tissue around his eyes and brow, which has permanently distorted the shape of this area for good; the pained, light's-too-bright squint.

He shuffles more than he did in his fighting heyday, and likes to take his time, but that's just fine because Matilda is in a patient mood this afternoon. She has a soft drink to keep her energised and is simply thankful to be somewhere else (the pair of them have been spending a lot of time at Charing Cross Hospital of late because Rocky's partner and Matilda's mother, Mandy, is battling cancer). 'This is where I used to fight,' Rocky tells his daughter as they approach a door.

To say this is where he used to fight is both factually correct and yet somehow offering only an abridged, child-safe version of events. It is true, of course, that Rocky used to box here, but it's true also to say that the venue has been elevated, both in his mind and mine, for reasons other than the simple fact he used to compete in its boxing ring. As I watch him enter the conference room, I know his mind isn't necessarily flooded with memories from fights – normal, routine fights – against the likes of Franky Moro or Phil Duckworth, two men he boxed here in 1985 and 1986 respectively. Nor is he recalling his rematch with Moro here in 1987. Rocky is, I suspect, thinking back to 14 March 1986, the night he faced Scotland's Steve Watt here. That was a fight. One hell of a fight, truth be told. But it was so much more than that. It would also be Watt's last.

The two men supporting Rocky this afternoon, Harry and John Holland, father and son, share many of the same memories and process them in the same order: Steve Watt tragedy followed by everything else. Likewise, this venue, formerly the old West Hotel, now one of many Ibis hotels, is as much an old stomping ground of theirs as it is Rocky's. It's their favourite West London haunt, in fact, the scene of many great fights, trove of so many precious memories, and the last time the three of them were united in this building the year was 1987.

The Hollands do most of the talking, and jog Rocky's

memory from time to time, but it's essentially a team affair. Always has been. Rocky did the fighting; the Hollands did the nurturing. They were in it together and it has been this way since Rocky, in and out of care homes from the age of seven, turned up at Harry's boxing gym in Chiswick as a thirteen-year-old calling himself 'Amilton and in need of a father figure. It's why they're back together.

'When Rocky fought here, we'd always have problems with forged tickets,' says Harry, kitted out in his finest black sports tracksuit, as if having come straight from the gym or, indeed, 1987. 'We had all sorts of complaints. Fellas would come up to me and say they'd paid for seats and there was someone else sat in their seat when they arrived. It was a bloody nightmare.'

He could laugh about it now.

'Nigel Benn used to buy tickets to see Rocky fight,' adds John. 'He loved him. All boxers loved him. He was a fighter's fighter.'

I turn to look at Rocky, still by his daughter's side, and he drops his eyes to the floor. He doesn't want to believe the stories. He's too humble and too dignified to ever dream of bathing in such glory. Moreover, Rocky, in this moment, has different images in his head. He's thinking not of packed crowds or Nigel Benn but of the scene that greeted him the day after his fight with Steve Watt, when Rocky took it upon himself to visit his opponent in hospital only to find a man in a coma with his hair shaved off and tubes connected to his head. *That's* the image he associates with this place. The rest is just wallpaper.

We enter the conference room, an expansive pink and purple floor space with purple neon lights running across the ceiling and walls, and all that's in the middle of the room is a closed suitcase, a number of stacked chairs and the odd table. 'The roof has all been modernised,' says Harry, exploring. 'They had chandeliers hanging there before.'

'The lighting's changed, certainly,' confirms his son.

Matilda skips around the room, drink still in hand, careful not to spill it, and throws her arms about. Rocky slowly paces behind her, but has no intention of catching up. He stares at the ceiling and the bright lights, then smiles at Harry.

'I think it could hold about fifteen hundred, but we got two thousand in here sometimes,' says Harry. 'There were two thousand most nights Rocky fought because of the forged tickets. You couldn't move. Eh, Rocky?'

Rocky again bows his head. Rather than elaborate, he gets closer to Matilda. 'This is where I used to fight,' he says, hand out in front. 'Right here.'

'I know,' his daughter replies. 'You said.'

Now out of earshot, distance from Rocky allows Harry the chance to really drum up some fanfare. 'Listen,' he says, 'if it wasn't for bloody Kirkland Laing, he,' pointing to the back of Rocky, 'would have been a world champ on guts alone. He was the most exciting fighter you'd ever see round here, fight after fight after fight, and I'm not just saying that because I was involved with him. The fight against Andy Furlong, for example...' Harry pauses to allow his son, John, to shake his head in disbelief. 'He's four rounds behind, he's cut over both eyes and the only reason the referee didn't stop it was because he was friendly with me. He came over and said, "Harry, he hasn't got much left, I'll leave it to you." I've said to him, "Rocky, it's the last round, we've spoken about this, get out there, finish this or your career's over." He went boom, boom, boom, had him down three times and stopped him. The guts that took. Can you imagine if someone said that to you? I know it would have broken me. That's the difference between us. His guts alone are the reason why everyone remembers him. I've had British champions, European champions and all sorts and when I see people they don't ask me about them. They always say, "How's Rocky?"'

As Rocky drifts and Harry waxes lyrical, a stuffy Eastern European woman in a tight-fitting suit, whose name-tag reads Adriana, yanks open the door and peeks inside the room. There is a clipboard in her hand and a perplexed look on her face. 'Excuse me,' she says, 'what are you doing in here?'

Rocky immediately looks the other way. He backtracks. Harry, though, offers his hand.

'My name's Mr Holland,' he says, 'Harry Holland. And this is my son John. You wouldn't know him, but this,' he points to the cowering figure on his right, 'is Rocky Kelly.'

Adriana looks the former boxer up and down. Her face remains blank.

'Rocky used to box here. He used to be on the TV in the eighties. He was a big star. We're just reminiscing.'

'We need to discuss,' says Adriana. 'We need to talk with our legal people and discuss logos in articles. You'll need approval for that first.'

'We're not looking to do anything now. This is history.'

'You should have got an appointment first. We don't just let people walk in and walk around the place.'

'No, it's okay,' says Harry, shaking his head. 'They told me to come down because in the future, if ever we promote again here, it's good to keep a good relationship.'

'We host some kickboxing events,' says Adriana, now apparently interested. 'The capacity with the boxing ring inside is around eight hundred with chairs.'

Harry scoffs at such an amount. 'I'm surprised,' he says. 'I thought it would be much more than that. We used to have fifteen hundred here.'

'Never!' Her clipboard is now gripped tighter than before. She's certain of it. 'The venue hasn't changed, it has just been refurbished.'

'I know. I'm just saying we used to get fifteen hundred in here.'

'You didn't.'

'No, we did,' says John, coming to his father's rescue. 'It was different in them days. Health and safety was different. We had fifteen hundred in here.'

'I've been working at this venue for ten years. The venue hasn't changed its capacity.'

'This is 1982, love.'

'Oh.'

'Along the back there'd be people standing, probably six or seven rows deep, and you can imagine how packed it was. It was the same against every wall. There might be eight hundred seats, but there'd be hundreds more standing.'

'Well, we can do eight hundred now. We have bars inside to provide refreshments. The kickboxing people like to have that. Maybe it's different logistics. The venue itself, without the ring, is twelve hundred. Obviously, depending on what you have around the ring, how many press you have, how many judges, how many other things, it all adds up.'

'I remember the fighters would change upstairs and come down in the lift,' says Harry, looking around. 'There were no bars in here in those days. We'd have drinks upstairs in the pub.'

'That's still here.'

'There's so much history to this place, you know. Years

ago, Rocky here had a fight with a man named Steve Watt and unfortunately he died. He was taken away from us too early.'

'Well, I'm sorry to hear that. But, really, you should have made an appointment.'

Adriana spins on her heels and leaves.

'Why did they call you Rocky?' asks Matilda.

'Because I was like Rocky, innit?' says her father, who then turns to me to add, 'She's seen the *Rocky* films but ain't really paid attention.'

'What about "The Explosive Rocky Kelly"?' I ask, referencing his memorable *nom de guerre*. 'Where did that come from?'

'When I used to see someone "go", I'd just charge into them and hit them with whatever I could. You just know when you've got them "going". You put pressure on them.'

'I put that name on his shorts because he's explosive,' says Harry. 'He explodes. He was an exciting fighter. That's our boy.'

Harry puts an arm around his boy and pulls him close.

'I used to love getting hit and going back for more. I didn't mind taking one or two to get close and dish my own out.'

'He had about forty amateur fights and then turned pro at eighteen, didn't you, Rocky?' says John.

'Yeah, that's right.'

'Bring back memories, Rocky?' says Harry.

'Yeah. I can't believe it.'

'Good memories, yeah?'

'Yeah. I've had some bad memories here, but mostly good. I've sold this place out, I've had my hand raised. I put smiles on people's faces, didn't I?'

'Absolutely. Did you hear her saying they can only get

eight hundred in here? Bollocks. You used to get double that. That's how popular you were.'

'I remember. The noise was deafening.'

It's silent now, though. Silent because Rocky isn't one for words or fancy descriptions, and silent because, unlike every one of the hotel guests who now frequent these premises, he knows what once occurred here. Not the fights but *the fight*.

Worst of all, Rocky remembers the words he said to Steve Watt the morning of their fight, having just both weighed in at the welterweight limit of ten stone seven pounds. 'Steve,' Rocky said that fateful day, looking his opponent straight in the eye, 'I'm willing to die for this.'

THE GOOD SON I

A red-rimmed triangular sign complete with an image of a strutting silhouette, situated not far from a series of white lines on the road, appears to have stumped a man from Youngstown, Ohio. He stops before the sign, unsure what to make of it, and then reads the words beneath it slowly and out loud: 'New... zebra... crossing... ahead.' He reads it a second time for good measure. Even slower this time. Just to make sure. 'What the hell does *that* mean?' asks Ray 'Boom Boom' Mancini, the former WBA (World Boxing Association) lightweight champion of the world, on a chilly October afternoon in Cannock, Staffordshire. 'Are there new zebras coming through here?'

Sensing his ill-placed intrigue and excitement at the prospect of witnessing an imminent stampede, I feel at liberty to explain the true meaning of the sign, ward him off waiting around any longer, and to instead use its power to slow down traffic and cross the road. So that's exactly what I do.

'So many things get lost in translation,' he says with a sigh as we walk towards Bar Sport, the venue in which a 'Gala Dinner Evening with Ray Mancini' will later take place. 'I've got to ask for the "loo" as well, right? You know, if I need to go...'

'I think toilet is okay,' I reply.

'And I've got to say "cheers" when someone helps me out?'

'You can if you want.'

'And if something's *really* great, I say it's "wicked"?'

Inside Bar Sport's Premier suite, Ray stands beside Scott Murray, the venue's owner and promoter, and takes a look around. The room, which will later host Mancini, the star, and hundreds of paying fans, appears set for a lavish wedding reception. There's a top table, numerous others facing it, and white tablecloths draped everywhere. There are also British and American flags hanging from the ceiling and a large screen erected at the back of the room, near the top table, on which highlights of Mancini's storied career will play. 'It's lovely,' Ray tells Scott in his best English accent. 'Lov-er-ly.'

It's better than 'wicked', I think to myself.

'We've got almost three hundred in tonight,' says Scott. 'You can probably squeeze a couple more tables in, but that's it.'

Happy with the set-up, Murray asks Mancini to settle down in a black chair outside the room and autograph a number of pictures and boxing gloves, which soon land in his lap. He does as he's told. Off comes his leather jacket, now hung over the back of his seat, and a variety of marker pens – black, gold and green – are caressed in his left hand.

'I fought my first six amateur fights as a southpaw but then my amateur trainer converted me,' he says. 'I got more use out of my left hand, the hook, the jab, uppercut, all from the left side.'

With this famous left hand, he signs dozens of printouts of his 1982 *Sports Illustrated* magazine cover, titled 'Boom Boom Booms', and some gold Everlast boxing gloves. The cover resonates most. It's an image of Mancini finishing a left hook against Ernesto España with an open-air stadium crowd and bright blue sky acting as a backdrop. 'It was in the middle of baseball season as well,' he says. 'I was very honoured by it.'

Moving images are soon to follow as Scott test-runs his highlights package on the big projector screen in the Premier Suite and on a smaller screen to the right of where Mancini sits signing gloves. It's a welcome distraction. He turns to look now and again. First up is footage of his 1984 WBA world lightweight title defence against fellow American Bobby Chacon. We're in round one. They're already unloading punches as though they're in short supply.

'Is it strange watching yourself?' a man in a suit asks.

'A little,' Ray says. 'I don't make a habit of it, if that's what you mean.'

As a fifty-four-year-old Mancini shakes out the cramp in his left wrist, the result of signing the first batch of gloves and photographs, a twenty-three-year-old version on screen smothers Chacon against the ropes.

'I know I didn't get the best of Bobby,' Ray says, almost apologetic in tone, taking no great pleasure from seeing someone he once admired get taken out in round three. 'Bobby was in his thirties, I was twenty-three. I had to make him fight at a twenty-three-year-old's pace. That's what I did and it took a toll on his body.' A replay of the finishing punches is shown on screen: Mancini, throwing both hands at the body and head of Chacon, never lets up; Chacon never goes down. 'Bobby liked to get you on the ropes and sucker-punch you. He always did. I kept him there. I didn't let him dictate. I didn't give him any space. But I love Bobby and I'd hate to think what sort of fight we'd have had if we were both at our best. It would have been a hard fifteen rounds.'

Bobby Chacon was known as 'Schoolboy' throughout his sixteen-year professional boxing career and went on to have sixty-seven pro fights. He won the WBC (World Boxing Council) world featherweight title in 1974 and the WBC world super-featherweight title in 1982. A fan favourite, during this time he waged career-shortening classics with the likes of Rafael 'Bazooka' Limón (four times), Rubén Olivares (three times), Cornelius Boza-Edwards (twice) and Alexis Argüello (mercifully, just once).

Chacon, now sixty-four, can hardly talk. He mumbles. He shuffles. He requires the assistance of carers. 'Schoolboy' has dementia pugilistica. He will die within twelve months of this interview.

'The last time I saw Bobby he was getting bad,' says Ray. 'He had a lot of wars, he didn't live right outside the ring and he blames himself for his wife's suicide [Valerie, his wife, unsuccessfully begged Bobby to stop boxing and so, the day before he fought Salvador Ugalde in 1982, she grabbed a rifle and shot herself]. Also, his son [Bobby Jr] got killed by gangs. He harmed himself for all that. He self-medicated. Look, we all had the opportunity to bang the bottle, bang the pipe or hit the needle, but I put my faith in God. That's how I got through it. You rely on your faith, you say your prayers and you gain strength from that.'

Ray has MRI scans done every year and will have another one this coming November. His only physical issues, he says, are to do with his wrists and shoulders, all of which show signs of arthritis, but he concedes old age could be just as responsible for that as his former profession. All in all, he feels good. 'My father said I heal good,' he says with a smirk. 'Seriously, though, I've spoken to enough neurologists and brain surgeons to know what does the damage and it's punishment taken over an extended period of time. Well, I only fought professionally for five and a half years. The guys who fight ten or fifteen years, guys like Tommy Hearns and Evander Holyfield, *they* suffer. Evander is a good guy but he won't know his own name five years from now. It's tragic. He might have made $300 million in the ring, but what good is it if you can't count it? Health is everything. The one thing I'm most proud of is the fact I can still spell "fight". So many guys can't. I hope and pray that will still be the case in ten years from now. We'll see. I don't worry about it.'

Today he looks and sounds great. The hair, once full and dark and often sloping down his neck, has thinned out and greyed, as is to be expected, but his general appearance remains much the same as it did in the eighties, much the same as it is in the old pictures he signs. He remains Fonzie-cool. There's a leather jacket slung over his chair and shiny stud earrings in his ears. A necklace, too. He also stays active, as if a fight's just around the corner. This morning he shadowboxed and skipped without a skipping rope in his hotel room while the television played. It's something he does most days. In fact, Ray has been skipping without a skipping rope ever since the peculiar art was taught to him by his father, Lenny, back in Youngstown in the seventies. Back then, Ray skipped sans rope out of necessity because the ceiling in the Mancini household was too low for him to use a rope inside. 'Just pretend,' said Lenny, a former pro fighter who once got within touching distance of a world title shot. 'It's all the same.' Now it's no longer unusual or strange, no longer anything to feel embarrassed about. So what if there's no rope in his hands. The act remains the same. 'You feel silly at first,' Ray explains, 'but it becomes natural over time. Also, if you're watching TV, you take your mind off the stupidity of it all. You take your mind to a different place.'

The next fight on screen is another quick one. It's Mancini's one-round dismissal of Johnny Torres in a non-title fight from 1983. This one grabs his complete attention. It's footage he hasn't seen for a long time and features a finish he's particularly fond of.

'Before this fight everyone was saying what a dangerous fight it was for me because he was a big, strong junior-welterweight,' he says. 'I saw him fight and thought he stands there and punches in front of you. I'll have some of that. I'd rather that than have him running away. After I knocked him out, I went over to Don Rickles, who was at ringside, and said, "Don, four tickets for tonight!"'

Mancini's infectious laugh is mimicked by a hyperactive bald-headed man named Shaun, who, we soon learn, is responsible for the night's photography. 'It will be as fast and as painless as possible, Ray,' he says.

'That's great,' replies Ray. 'Thank you.'

'Not many I've wanted to meet as much as you.'

'You're too kind.'

Shaun dumps a pile of glossy A4 photographs on the seat beside Ray, in the hope they'll be signed, and then switches his attention to the screen in the corner of the room by the bar.

'I was watching the Livingstone Bramble fights the other night,' he says. 'I think you were robbed.'

Mancini shrugs but continues signing. 'The second fight, I thought I beat him. In the first fight I was beating him but it wasn't my night. He caught me. My body betrayed me. I thought I out-punched him in the rematch.'

'And the [Héctor] Camacho fight as well...'

'Oh, Camacho, man,' says Ray, 'that was a good fight, not a great fight, but I beat him. All he did was run. Mills Lane, the referee, said, "Look, I'm not going to second-guess the judges, that would be bullshit, but safe to say if Mancini wasn't in there tonight there'd have been no fight."'

His 1989 WBO (World Boxing Organization) world light-welterweight title snoozer with Camacho is next on screen.

'I just didn't have my timing,' he says, glumly, eyes on the television. 'I'm falling short, I'm reaching. He's got nothing on his jabs but I can't cut off the ring. They wanted a twenty-two-foot ring, we wanted an eighteen, so they settled on twenty. I said, "So what?" It *is* a big ring, though. You've got to chase him down. Too far out, too far out...'

He'd lose a split-decision to Camacho that March night, one debated for years afterwards. Boxer versus brawler, it depended on your preference; a rusty Mancini forced the pace but Camacho made him jig to his beat. Ray blamed the hair. 'I had the mullet thing going on,' he says. 'That's what was happening at that time. But the problem with hair like that is every time you get hit, the hair flies back. The judges pick up on that.'

Ray gets back to signing gloves. The images on screen are the cause of too much frustration. It's not good for him. The mood becomes serious. 'Was it "Harry" I was supposed to be signing?' he asks no one in particular. A shrug follows.

'Who was the best fighter you ever fought?' I ask, keen to avert his gaze from the clips of him chasing an elusive Camacho for twelve rounds.

'Alexis Argüello, hands down.'

Soon Ray alternates between signing Shaun's latest batch of photographs and revelling in images from his WBA world lightweight title win over Arturo Frias in 1982. The night it all came true. The night Lenny, his father, had never been prouder. The night it was done and dusted inside three minutes. 'Not too many world titles are won in the first round,' says Mancini. 'I'm flattered when people say it was the best one-round fight in history. I'm so honoured by that.'

His proud old man, Lenny Mancini, a leading contender on the brink of a title shot at lightweight, was drafted for the Second World War and wounded in Metz in 1944. He'd fight again, after recovering from his injuries, but was never the same, never quite as intense, and Father Time ensured he never received the world title chance he craved.

As one dream faded, however, another grew and Ray, his son, would eventually adopt the same moniker as his father, that of 'Boom Boom', and go in search of the one thing that escaped Lenny Mancini – the world lightweight championship. For a middle-class kid raised in a decent neighbourhood, this would become Ray's so-called righteous reason for fighting and was a goal he fulfilled in 1982.

Anyway, those were the good times, the moments to savour, the moments he doesn't mind replaying on a grim Thursday afternoon in the West Midlands. But for every Frias or Chacon or Torres, there's a question about defeats to Camacho or Bramble or reminders of something much, much worse.

'Where's Scott?' Mancini asks in a panic as he looks at the

screen and then looks away just as quickly. His red sweater tightens around his neck. Sweat patches immediately show beneath his armpits.

'I don't know,' I say, distracted, staring at one of the half-signed pictures of Mancini on the coffee table.

'This is awful. We need to get him here *now*!'

I look up to see grainy footage of Mancini's 1982 fight with Duk Koo Kim on screen.

'We can't have this playing!' says Ray, rising from his chair. 'Where's Scott?'

Not a moment too soon, Scott arrives on the scene, clocks what is showing on the projector, muffles an involuntary yelp and darts into the Premier Suite to change it. But Mancini, face pale, as if having spotted a ghost at the end of his bed, is seemingly unable to stop shaking. 'That can't happen again,' he says, retreating to his seat. 'Can you imagine how bad that would be if it started playing while people are eating their dinner tonight? It would be terrible.'

Murray returns a minute later to apologise.

'Scott, come on, that has *got* to be taken out,' says Ray.

'I've removed it completely,' says Scott. 'I'm so sorry. It was just a general highlight reel of fights, that's all.'

'I know nothing was meant by it. It's nobody's fault. But it can't happen again.'

Earlier that day, I joined Ray and Scott and Ray's wife, Tina, for afternoon tea and soup at their hotel overlooking a Cannock A-road. During the course of our conversation, I referenced an article published by the local *Express and Star* newspaper as part of the promotion for the evening's event, in which Mancini was described in the opening paragraph as, 'The boxer who was involved in a ring tragedy that led to world title fights being reduced to twelve rounds...' There was no mention of his father, no mention of Arturo Frias and their one-round epic, and the following paragraphs merely added layers of detail to what had already been established from the offset; Ray Mancini, a former world champion, had once killed a man in the boxing ring and was now visiting Cannock to tell all.

The life in Ray's eyes faded. He played with the remnants of his carrot soup.

'They try to sensationalise it,' he said, despondently. 'It doesn't happen so much in America any more, but I guess they still do that here. I ignore it. I like to think I had a pretty good career. I won the title for my father, defended it five times. Was I defined by that fight? Perhaps. Is that one I'm best known for? Well, if it is, that's a shame. That's unfortunate. But I'm not going to get angry or start calling people out. I understand it.'

'That article was written by a reporter who has no knowledge of our sport,' said Murray. 'He has put Ray's name into Google and mentioned whatever he sees at the top of the page. They're just looking for an angle. It's disgraceful, really.'

'They even used a picture of that Kim fight on the poster for this event,' Ray added.

'I was really sorry about that,' said Scott.

'I understand. You didn't mean anything by it. But I won't sign anything with that picture.'

'We've changed it now.'

'I know. But what I'm saying is if that's what I'm best known for my career wasn't worth a whole lot.' Mancini shrugged his shoulders, then sipped from a mug of pomegranate tea. 'I don't answer questions about it any more simply because the book and the documentary came out,' he continued, referring to *The Good Son*, book written by Mark Kriegel, documentary directed by Jesse James Miller. 'People say to me, "Well, what about the Kim fight?" I say, "Have you read the book?" They say, "Yeah, yeah." So I say, "Have you seen the documentary?" They say, "Yeah, of course." Then I say, "Well, that's all I've got to say on the matter. Read the book or watch the documentary and you've got your answers." That's why I did them, so there was nothing left to answer. Together, they answer every question.'

Selfishly speaking, this is hardly what you want to hear when sat with a notebook full of questions, many of which pertain to the very thing the interviewee would rather not discuss, and a Dictaphone ready to pounce. At best, it rouses feelings of frustration and disappointment; at worst it brings on introspection. Why am I doing this? Why do I want to grill this man about an incident that clearly distresses him? Does the fact I've decided to copy his choice of a pomegranate tea constitute enough common ground to enable him to open up and dish the dirt? Will he soon hate me? Stuff like that.

I've read the book, I've watched the documentary, but still I'm going to probe, I decide. It would be gutless and hypocritical to bail at this stage. After all, I've watched the fourteen rounds that proved to be Duk Koo Kim's last. I sat through it, eyes wide open, marvelling at the bravery on display, and it would be wrong of me, therefore, to act like it doesn't exist within the context of Ray Mancini's career. Regrettably, his story isn't complete without Kim. The two men are, for better or worse, inextricably linked.

Later, as he signs photographs and gloves, he receives another reminder of this when coming across a picture from the Kim fight in the pile he's in the process of wading through. On discovering it, colour immediately drains from his face. His posture loses its form and seems to deflate. He sinks into the chair. His pen drops from his hand on to the table.

'I can't sign that,' he says, pointing to the picture. 'I just can't. I'm sorry.'

The image, one of Mancini and Kim throwing punches at Caesars Palace, had originally been used on the Bar Sport poster to promote the evening's event, and Ray had already made it quite clear he disapproved. But this was now too much. Shaun, the photographer, gets wind of Ray's malaise and is quick to offer an apology. 'Sorry about that, Ray,' he says. 'I didn't even realise it had got in there.'

Ray smiles back. 'No, it's okay,' he says. 'Don't apologise. I understand.'

'I specifically said to them not to send any pictures that had anything to do with that fight. I'm going to kick their arse now.'

'No, it's fine. You wouldn't believe the amount of people who come up to me with pictures from that fight. I understand, you've got to take the shot, but I ain't doing it. I don't blame people. Sometimes they don't even know. You have to tell them. That's the worst.'

Shaun puts both hands together in a praying motion and moves closer to his hero. 'Ray,' he says, 'on my eyes, I apologise. I didn't mean anything by it.'

'I know you didn't. Please don't apologise. You didn't upset me at all.'

'I had a guy make them for me and I specifically said to him I didn't want anything to do with that particular fight. I'm fuming!'

In a rage, Shaun takes the image in question and proceeds to rip it in half, then quarters and then into smaller and smaller bits until it is no more. 'There you go, Ray,' he says, 'it's gone!'

No video clips, no pictures, no reminders, Mancini's stance on the Kim fight is by now totally clear. Yet here's the confusing part. As he leaves Bar Sport, later to return for his big night, Ray walks down a set of stairs, points to the original event poster on the wall, featuring an image from the Kim fight, and says to Scott Murray, 'Could you send me a copy of that poster, Scott? I'd like to show it to the family.'

Unsure whether he's being tested, having seen Ray's earlier reaction to the very same image, Murray uncomfortably fidgets, before replying, 'Sure, Ray, but do you want me to mask out the picture?'

'Boom Boom' shakes his head. 'No, leave it,' he says. 'It's fine.'

5

THE CROWDPLEASER II

At seven years of age, Hamilton Kelly already had a strict routine in place, one that consisted of him getting up in the morning, walking to his mother's bedroom and proceeding to wake up both his mother and his older brother, Tommy, who was born mentally handicapped and slept in the same bed.

Most of the time this process ran smoothly and without incident. His mother was usually groggy, having been kept up most of the night, and Tommy could often be unpredictable, but nothing ever flustered Hamilton, nor made him resent his role.

Along with his older sister Diane, this was his lot, his family, and it had been that way ever since his mother snatched him from a barber's in Liverpool and out of the arms of his Trinidadian father and took him to west London. His parents' relationship was a volatile one at the best of times, but the sudden separation and 'kidnapping', as Hamilton describes it, came as something of a surprise. One minute he was enjoying time with his father at the barbershop and the next he was out of Liverpool and now in London, blinded by the bright lights, enrolling in a new school and being bullied by pupils for his scouse accent. Hamilton, scouse and mixed race, couldn't understand it. He struggled to adjust.

The one consistency he had in his life was this morning routine. *Get out of bed and wake Mum and Tommy.* It was his job, his role in the household, and he knew nothing else. So he did it, time and time again, until one day he struggled to wake his mum from her slumber.

'Mum! Mum! Mum!' he said. 'It's time to get up!'

There was no movement, no sign of her rising, and Tommy and Hamilton innocently assumed she was enjoying a deep sleep.

She was, in fact, dead.

Anti-depressant pills had 'done her in', Rocky believes, the cause of death a brain haemorrhage, and that morning, as he looked into the whites of her eyes, soon to be forever haunted by the image, he wondered all sorts of things: *How? Why? What now?* He was just seven years of age. He had a mentally handicapped brother by his side. He had no answers. All he knew was that his mother, the person supposed to guide him through life, was dead in his arms.

'Have you seen pictures of Steve Watt?' Rocky asks me out of the blue.

We're now free of the old conference room, back out in the corridor, sat on a dark red leather sofa, but memories of the scene remain. The carpet, the lights, the stacked chairs, the suitcase. Memories of the chandeliers. Memories of the battles. The sounds, the smells, the violence. Images of death are never far from Rocky's mind.

'Only in the fight,' I reply.

'So I fought this geezer and he was really hard. He had a right face on him and we were saying words to each other. We were two proud young men. Two strong, fit, proud men. But, the day after, I went to see him in hospital and it was dreadful. He had half his hair shaved off and he had all these tubes in his head. He had black eyes, lumps all over his face. I thought, fucking hell... you don't see the damage you do to the people you fight. He was in a bad way. I couldn't believe it.'

Rocky wipes a tear with his forearm and then makes for the toilet. He'll be back in a few minutes, I'm told, which leaves just enough time for Harry and John Holland, his wingmen, to rewind and fill in some of the blanks. Wasting not even a second, I'm informed Steve Watt first fought Rocky Kelly in the semi-finals of the ABAs (Amateur Boxing Association) and that Watt went into the bout as a heavy favourite on account of the fact he'd already fought three times that day and stopped every one of his opponents within the distance. A big puncher, then, most assumed he'd have his way with the primitive Kelly. Harry Holland, though, had other ideas. He concocted a game plan that would see his man flip the script on Watt and instead of bull-rushing him, as was his custom, he'd use underrated boxing skills, skills he'd honed under the tutelage of Holland, to take the play away from Watt and outbox him, which he did, winning the fight on points.

'The fight with Steve Watt was a tremendous fight,' recalls John, 'and there was that little bit of rivalry between them because of it. Everyone said Steve had the pro style to beat Rocky and their careers ran parallel as pros. People expected they'd one day box again.'

Kelly turned professional in October 1981 and Watt followed suit in February 1983. By this time, Watt had heard about the good job Harry Holland was doing with Kelly and decided to approach him with a view to working with him. He wanted Harry to be his manager. So they met, swapped ideas and discussed a plan, but, in the end, Watt decided against going with Holland because he believed his allegiance with Kelly would prove a conflict of interest. Second fiddle wasn't an option for him, not when about to embark on a pro career. He wanted to be in the driving seat. 'But he was wrong,' says Holland, decades later. 'What you do is take them different ways. If they have to meet for, say, a world title, so be it, but you only do that when the time is right and the price is right. I would have guided Rocky and Steve away from each other.'

There's a rueful look on Holland's face. He calls that meeting an 'evil twist of fate', and says that if Watt had trusted him just that little bit more he would likely never have crossed paths with Rocky Kelly for a second time. If only. As it happened, Watt won eleven of his first twelve professional fights, including a fifth-round stoppage of Tommy McCallum for the Scottish Area welterweight title, and was then reacquainted with Kelly, his old amateur rival, on 14 March 1986.

Rocky, at this stage, had packed a fair amount into his own twenty-five-bout career. He'd lost four times, won the rest, and lifted the Southern Area welterweight title in February 1984 with a decision win over Chris Sanigar at the Royal Albert Hall. He'd also unsuccessfully challenged for the British welterweight title when coming unstuck against Kostas Petrou in nine rounds in April 1985. But, undeterred, he was hopeful he'd get another shot at the belt and was told a win over Steve Watt in an eliminator bout would be just the ticket.

Rocky took to training camp with a renewed bounce in his step. There'd be no disappointment this time round, he told himself. He was going to whip his body into career-best shape, defeat Steve Watt in their eliminator and then do the same to the British welterweight champion Kirkland Laing. A clear schedule in mind, he trained for the Watt fight in Tenerife alongside Harry Holland, and stayed true to his word. 'He was always fit but that was the ultimate,' Holland purrs. 'As I was rubbing him down one day, someone walked in and said, "Fucking hell, Rocky, you're like a racehorse." They were the exact words I had in my head, too. He was shiny like a racehorse.'

Rocky, now back with us following his toilet break, smiles at the description. Full of pride, he remembers being in that shape once. He remembers weighing ten stone seven. He remembers being that racehorse, that machine. But he also knows time has softened both his edges and his mentality. If in doubt, a doting glance the way of Matilda, now sleeping on the arm of the sofa, offers all the evidence needed.

Back to the racehorse. When the time came to confront Steve Watt at the weigh-in on the morning of the fight, Harry told Rocky to arrive suited and booted and to carry the appearance of a champion. So he did. He always did as he was told. Steve, on the other hand, arrived wearing a tracksuit. It was considered a sign. A sign one was comfortable and one still had work to do. 'Steve had to boil down whereas Rocky never really had a problem making weight,' says John. 'He was a welterweight his whole career.'

John's father nods in agreement. 'We always used to get Rocky down to the weight in advance,' he says. 'The thing is, Steve Watt's trainer always seemed to try and bring him down a weight lower. Steve Watt was very, very strong at middleweight. He was stopping them all. Then he was a light-middleweight stopping them all. As a pro, he started off at light-middleweight and then they brought him down to welterweight. I still think the dehydration from making weight had something to do with *it*.'

The two fighters weighed in, both registering a weight of ten stone seven pounds, and after shaking hands Rocky uttered the immortal line which now won't go away: 'Steve, I'm willing to die for this.'

Twenty-nine years later, the three men on the sofa, Rocky, Harry and John, take a deep breath, almost in unison, and lower their heads. 'At the time,' says Harry, 'the hairs on the back of my neck stood up and I thought, flipping hell, I wouldn't like to be fighting him. He wasn't being horrible saying that, he was just so determined and confident. It showed how much he wanted it.'

'After the fight that was taken out of context and some of the Watt family reacted badly to it,' adds John. 'But he made no reference to Steve dying.'

Kelly nods. 'It was a grudge match, me and Steve Watt,' he says. 'We had that history and he always thought he was better than me. He was good in his manor and I was good in my manor. We fought to prove who was the best.'

Watching the contest on DVD nearly thirty years later feels strange, not least because fights such as the one produced by Kelly and Watt are such a rarity these days. Consider, for example, the fact there were no lulls or rounds used to 'feel out' the opponent's style, commonplace nowadays. Appreciate, too, the fact that fighters like Kelly and Watt didn't come to win on points or minimise risk. Conversely, they didn't feel victory was theirs until they'd made a tangible impression on the other man's body and soul. Winning rounds wasn't enough. They punched whenever they were in position to punch and took aim at even the slightest hint of target. There were no second thoughts. Nothing was weighed up or contemplated. It just happened. It was, I guess, as pure as professional fighting is ever likely to get; two men *truly* fighting as opposed to hiding behind the literal definition of boxing, that is to hit and not get hit, and saving themselves for another (pay) day.

'That was a proper fight,' Rocky recalls. 'I remember the referee slapping us on the head in the second round because we were close together, but, other than that, he never got involved. He just stood back and let us get on with it. You see some referees getting in there and making a nuisance of themselves, but he didn't do that once. We didn't need him. We didn't hit the ropes at all in the fight, either. We just stood there together in the middle of the ring. There was no quarter given.'

Up to the midway point in the fight, they'd operated at the same pace, in the same area of the ring – the middle – and had thrown there or thereabouts the same amount of leather. However, by the sixth round, there were signs, albeit only subtle ones, that Kelly's physical strength and athleticism was beginning to tell. He'd land shots on Watt and then budge the Scot immediately after, either with his shoulder or elbow, an act of dominance that let him build momentum, get his opponent on the retreat and also create space for a follow-up attack. Watt didn't have the same luxury. He'd land punches, of course, and rattle off some lovely combinations to head and body, but wouldn't then have the physicality to flee the scene or move Kelly away from him. This meant that no matter how quick his hands were, and how technical his boxing was, he would always remain in punching range and taste a little of whatever Kelly had to offer. There was, for Watt, no escape.

There were no knockdowns, nor were there any major flash points where one man appeared hurt by the other. It just wasn't that kind of fight. Both landed plenty, there's no question about that, but neither packed the power to dislodge the other from their senses or end the fight prematurely. A shame too in many ways because a lot can be said for the benefits of fights cut short by a big puncher. At least then the man on the receiving end is spared a prolonged beating. The fight is over in an instant. But Kelly and Watt were always likely to go the long haul, destined to keep punching one another until the final bell sounded and they were ripped apart. Sometimes those are the worst kind of fights.

'Rocky was two rounds in front on the scorecards going into the last round, but you couldn't be sure of that at the time,' says Harry, the main man in Kelly's corner that night. 'I've watched it over and over again to see if there's any deterioration in Steve before he stops him. But the round before he's turning Rocky, grabbing him by the elbows, messing him about. So, no, there were no signs.'

With two minutes gone in the tenth and final round, it happened. Exhaustion caught up with Watt and he found himself nailed by a Kelly left–right hook combination, which, rather than hurt him, knocked him off balance. Kelly swiftly followed with two more swings, one of which was a left hook to the body that sent Watt to the ropes, undoubtedly in pain, before he ran after his wounded opponent, threw a right hook, a left hook, turned him towards the ropes on the far side of the ring, and then hit Watt with another left and right hook, the last of which caught him slack-jawed and almost spun his head around. They were both now on autopilot; Watt surviving, Kelly finishing. As Watt sagged to the ropes for a second time, this one far worse, his head lolled, Kelly continued hitting him and referee Sid Nathan stopped the fight.

'The referee had to give him every chance in that tenth round,' says Harry. 'With hindsight, you could say he should have stopped it two punches before, but not on the night. It's a close fight and he could possibly turn it around. He had to give him every chance. Rocky never had him down. He staggered him against the ropes. He stopped him on his feet.'

'Sid Nathan wasn't in late,' agrees John. 'He punished himself for it, but he never did anything wrong. Steve was protesting. He didn't want to be stopped.'

The stoppage, which came at two minutes and seven seconds of the last round, seemed well timed if not perfect (it rarely is). Nathan got between them at the right moment, having given Watt the benefit of the doubt he deserved in a competitive fight, and called it off when less compassionate referees may have waited for the inevitable knockout. Nathan didn't. He got in there fast.

Fight over, Rocky Kelly jumped into the arms of Harry Holland, his trainer and father figure, and immediately felt his legs dissolve. He could hardly stand. He too had nothing left.

'As it ends, and he's the winner, he collapses in my arms,' says Harry. 'You see it on tape.'

'I never thought you knew that,' says Rocky.

'He,' pointing to Rocky beside him, 'wins, he's exhausted, he collapses, but he's okay. This meant so much to Steve

Watt as well and all of a sudden he's lost. He's lost the fight, he's lost his shot at the British title, and he's lost everything he believes in. That happens in a split-second for him. All of that emotion could have affected his brain. Accidents happen when fighters go beyond the call of duty, not just physically, but mentally and emotionally, too. Steve went to that place that night.'

'I had a bit of a premonition the night before,' says Rocky. 'I knew something was going to happen. That's why I said I was willing to die. Maybe I thought it was going to be me. I just had a feeling this wasn't going to be a normal boxing match.'

It was perfectly normal at first. Watt returned to his stool under his own steam and was even greeted and commiserated by Kelly. But then a vacant look came over the Scotsman and he slid down from his stool on to the canvas. Kelly, not far from his adversary, took one look at him and knew things had taken a drastic turn for the worse. 'I saw the same thing I saw when my mum died all those years ago,' he says. 'I saw something in his eyes. I knew there was something wrong with him.'

It's again too much for Rocky. His eyes well up and he uses a second toilet break to compose himself. This time I'm not sure whether it's the memory of the look on his mother's face or the memory of the look on Watt's face that gets to him. Most likely it's both.

'Rocky was the first one to say he'd collapsed,' remembers Harry. 'As soon as I heard that, something hit me and, I hate to say it, I immediately thought the worst. I don't know why. It was like a sixth sense or something. People had been knocked out and collapsed before. It didn't necessarily mean they would die. But I knew it wasn't going to end well. The terrible thing is there were no paramedics in those days. All that was required was that you had a stretcher. So we just put him on a bloody stretcher.'

Steve Watt was taken to Charing Cross Hospital on the Friday night and underwent surgery for the removal of a blood clot on the brain. After the operation, Rocky summoned the courage to go and visit his opponent and pay his respects. He couldn't believe the damage his fists had done. 'Rocky visiting Steve was all his own doing,' says Harry. 'People told him to stay away as it might not be safe. Steve had brothers and tensions were high. But Rocky just wanted to see him and speak to him.'

On the evening of Monday 17 March 1986, Steve Watt, twenty-eight, passed away from injuries sustained in his non-title fight. The coroner ruled cause of death to have been an acute bleed from a severed vein at the base of the skull and the reaction was one of horror from most sections of the British media. Those who wanted a total ban of the sport were now, they thought, justified in making such calls, while BBC's *Grandstand* shelved any plans they had to show the fight that weekend.

A guilt-ridden Kelly, protected from the public outcry by Harry, did the right thing. He attended Steve's funeral, against the advice of others, and bravely said goodbye in the presence of the Watt family and loved ones. That soothed him somewhat. It provided comfort.

More comfort was to follow once an investigation into the death was launched and it came to light Watt possessed a skull so abnormally thin that if it had been picked up by an MRI scan beforehand he'd have never been allowed to box; during the autopsy numerous scars from previous brain bleeds were discovered; he was, they said, an accident waiting to happen.

'You know when your brain is sitting in the jelly, his skull was a fraction of the size of Rocky's,' explains Harry. 'So his brain was being knocked all over the place whenever he got into the ring.'

'He'd been hit with all sorts all over his fucking head,' adds Rocky, sombrely. 'He was just that sort of fighter. Brave. Tough.'

'He should never have been boxing. These days an MRI would have picked it up in seconds.'

'I got a scan before that fight.'

'No, you didn't,' says Harry, putting his hand on Rocky's shoulder. 'They only brought them in *after* that fight.'

'That's what brought about the mandatory MRI scans,' says John. 'On the Sunday it was on the front pages of newspapers and something had to be done.'

It took Rocky six months to make sense of what happened to Steve Watt and then consider getting back in the ring and boxing again. It wasn't that he ever doubted his ability to do so, or even questioned whether he wanted to do it, more that he wanted to do it right, in the correct frame of mind, and didn't want his recent momentum to go to waste. After all, he was now about to fight for the British welterweight title again. There was a lot at stake.

'Rocky had to get over that,' says Harry. 'It was terrible. We had to both ask ourselves if we wanted to carry on.'

'Nah,' says Rocky, 'if it was going to happen to me, it was going to happen to me. I couldn't do nothing about it. There was no point being scared or worried. I just had to put it to the back of my mind and get on with things.'

It was in some ways easier for Rocky than others because his boxing career was one forever steeped in folklore and fantasy. It started with the name: Rocky. More than just an obvious ring sobriquet and an indication of style, this name symbolised a very distinct alter-ego and character, one Harry would encourage in an attempt to convince his fighter that the stark reality of both boxing and life was never much fun.

'What suited him was that it was all like a film to Rocky,' explains Harry. 'We made a decision for it to be like that from the start. His whole boxing career was like a film and he was a character in the film. I let him believe that because it helped in that moment. The *Rocky* films were dramatic and there were ups and downs and tragedies, and we took that approach with Rocky's career. Yes, a tragedy happened, but it was in the film that was his life.'

The Rocky story rolled into its next sequel, yet the star of the franchise, he of the title, remembers very few scenes. 'We had one fight after and fought some black geezer, didn't we?' asks Kelly.

Harry frowns. 'No,' he says, 'you had quite a few fights after that.'

'After Steve Watt?'

'Yeah.'

'No, I didn't.'

'You did. The first one was Mark Mills. Then you boxed Tony Brown, which was "Fight of the Year" in 1986, and that was an eliminator for the British title.'

'Oh, yeah, I remember now,' says Rocky.

'And you fought Kirkland Laing. Remember?'

Rocky nods.

'He had great fights afterwards, don't get me wrong,' says Harry, 'but his pinnacle was Steve Watt. The way his body was, the way he was mentally, he'd have beaten most in Britain that night. He was never quite the same after that.

He was still exciting and still one hell of a fighter, but that little edge wasn't quite there.'

'I didn't really want to retire, but I lost something,' admits Rocky. 'It just went from me.'

All in all, Kelly boxed a further eight times after the Watt tragedy, winning five of them, losing two and drawing one. He received his long overdue second shot at the British title in November 1987, only to find himself stopped by the enigmatic Kirkland Laing inside five rounds. The defeat rankles Kelly and Holland to this day, for they remain convinced the fight was halted prematurely and that Rocky, renowned for his ability to come on strong late, would have found a way to get to Laing in the closing stages. Who knows? What we do know, for sure, is there would be no major title for Rocky Kelly. He'd fall short in two British title attempts and then lose to Gary Jacobs in a Commonwealth title shot in February 1989. 'It chokes me really because he deserves to have been a world champion,' says Harry. 'I've never known anyone more gutsy in my life. If ever a man deserved one, it was him.'

All out of opportunities, Kelly had his last fight, a draw with Winston Wray, in September 1989. At twenty-six, he'd never box again.

'It was really hard,' he says, twenty-six years on. 'Boxing was my life – it's all I had. It saved me. You make so many friends in boxing and it's the people I miss. We were like one big family. Sometimes I thought about coming back.'

'He thought about it all the time,' Harry interjects. 'He got offers from the unlicensed circuit. It would have broken my heart if he'd come back and did that. But he never did.'

'They can't fight, can they?'

'No, you would have been demeaning yourself.'

'That's what I thought.'

'Yes, he retired at twenty-six, but, remember, he started at eighteen,' says Harry. 'He had eight years of hard fights.'

'Also,' says Kelly, 'I had my first child at fifteen. It was just different, man. It was hard. You've got to try and fit everything in, haven't you? My boxing career always came before anything. But I hurt a lot of people while doing it, like my family, my kids.'

Harry puts an arm around Rocky and John tenderly touches him on his knee. They sense their boy is suddenly consumed by regret and act to provide necessary comfort and reassurance. It's a sweet gesture, one which shows how much the two men care.

'He gave everything away,' says John. 'If Rocky had a tenner, he wouldn't want it in his pocket, he'd give it to you. That's him. Whenever Rocky fought, he treated the people around him. He was too generous. You didn't hurt anyone in your family. You gave everything away.'

'I did,' says Rocky. 'I didn't want it.'

'I always got him the best I could,' says Harry, who reckons Kelly would have made £2,000 for the Watt fight pre-tax and other deductions. 'It's just a shame Rocky didn't come around a little later because he would have made a lot more money.'

'As soon as Rocky got his money, he'd go straight down the care home to see Tommy, his brother, and he'd put a load of money there,' adds John. 'For years and years you couldn't get hold of Rocky on a Saturday because he'd take Tommy out of the home and to the pictures. They probably watched the latest film twenty times in a month.'

'I still take him out now,' Rocky says, smiling. 'But he doesn't know where he is or what's going on. It's like being out with a dummy. He just sits there and eats and eats.'

DOG ROUNDS

Parentless for much of his life, it was boxing and its extended family that created, nurtured and was ultimately responsible for Rocky. It was boxing, also, that blackened him with a ring tragedy and numerous fights in which he endured sustained punishment. This much is undeniable. He knows it, too. At one stage, he even stands and asks me to press his ribs, so proud is he of the time he had them broken in a 1982 'Fight of the Year' with Gary Knight, a fight which, I'm told, set the record for the most amount of 'nobbins' (coins) thrown into a British ring following a contest. Five hundred quid found its way into the Bloomsbury Centre ring that night, to be split by the pair, but Rocky no doubt paid the price. 'My ribs have been like that ever since,' he says. 'He did that to me in the first round.' A hard, resistant mass has formed on Kelly's ribs and he claims to no longer get any sensation in that area. It is, to him, merely a battle scar. No big deal.

A bigger deal, to me at least, is the long-lasting effect the many punches he received during the course of his crowd-pleasing eight-year professional career may have had on his memory, his speech and his long-term brain functionality. Unfortunately, there's no escaping such thoughts, not when sat opposite him, listening to him talk. And though he's delightfully childlike in his innocence, I start to question how much of this is due to his character, be it Rocky or Peter Pan, and how much of it is due to some kind of regression. 'I had to take a lot of punches because that was my style,' he says. 'I feel all right, though. Some people think I'm punchy – and they think the punches have affected me – but I don't.'

Harry and John are quick to leap to his defence.

'Rocky spoke like this when he was fifteen,' says Harry. 'No disrespect to him, but he has *always* been that way. I'm not the brightest person, Rocky ain't the brightest person, and we make mistakes when we talk. People misinterpret that and think he's punchy.'

'I came down to London from Liverpool and all of a sudden I'm a cockney geezer. I didn't get taught my words – these long words. I get very confused. It took me time to learn to pronounce my words properly. I've got them worked out in my brain but it takes a bit of time for me to say them. I'm not punchy, this is the way I've always been.'

'Added to that,' says Harry, 'he also had a bit of a drink problem, which I hope he doesn't mind me saying.'

Rocky shakes his head. He doesn't mind.

'He's over that now, but that affects people.'

'It's true.'

'When we went on a plane to Scotland to fight Dave Douglas,' says John, 'he said to my dad, "There's something following us out there." He looked out the window and pointed and my dad said, "It's the wing, Rocky, you fucking idiot." So, if he's punchy now, he was definitely punchy back then, too.'

All three of them laugh together.

'He has always been like that,' says Harry. 'I saw Chris Sanigar, his old opponent, one day in Hammersmith and I said to Rocky, "Look, there's Chris Sanigar," and he said, "Where?" I pointed to him. He's gone over there and is talking to a kid who is probably seventeen or eighteen, who's with Chris, and he's going, "Hello Chris, how are you?" I shouted out, "Not him, you clown!" But that's him. That's why we love him.'

Rocky doesn't care what people think and likes to downplay his achievements. He describes himself as a 'normal person' now, as if aware he was previously playing a part, and says he quite likes it. 'I'm still well known round this manor, but not as much now,' he concedes. 'I've got so many friends in boxing, but I don't remember their names. I don't know how you remember all the names, Harry.'

'Just remember the important ones, mate.'

'Like you.'

Harry kisses Rocky on his forehead. 'We're family. So is she.'

Harry's index finger is directed the way of Matilda, Rocky's ten-year-old, who wakes on the arm of the sofa and rubs her eyes.

'She's my youngest one,' says Rocky, who also fathered two children while in care; Tasha and Jermaine; he was just fifteen when Tasha was born. 'The problem is, when I was boxing, I couldn't really spend a lot of time with them. I was a kid myself. So I don't really know them. I mean, I know them now, but I don't know them the way I wish I knew them.'

'You always looked after them, Rocky,' reassures Harry.

'But I don't really know them, Harry. I love them, but they don't really love me. I haven't got a bond like you and John have.'

'*She* loves you,' says Harry, pointing at Matilda.

'She loves me because I'm with her all the time. But I've seen these two,' Rocky points at the men either side of him, 'together for years and years and they're still together. I don't have that bond with my kids. I don't really know them.'

Matilda goes and sits by her father. She then rolls her eyes.

'I'm never going to leave this one, though.'

6

THE GOOD SON II

What's a difference of three rounds? Not much, you might think, but a hell of a lot can happen in nine minutes. Bayern Munich striker Robert Lewandowski can score five goals in nine minutes, Red Rum overtook Crisp to win the 1973 Grand National in nine minutes, and 'Marvelous' Marvin Hagler and Thomas 'Hitman' Hearns were able to create arguably the greatest fight in boxing history within that time. Nine minutes, therefore, especially in boxing, can be the difference between winning and losing, the difference between life and death. 'The dog rounds,' says the former fighter sat opposite me. 'That's what I called the last three rounds. I called 'em the dog rounds because they'd bring out the dog in you.'

Today championship fights take place over twelve rounds, but, back in the eighties when Ray Mancini was WBA world lightweight champion, they were decided over fifteen. He preferred it that way, too. It gave him more time to pace himself, rev his engine and claw back any points deficit. It also, he says, distinguished the champions from the mere contenders, for if you couldn't do the business over the fifteen-round distance, the full forty-five minutes, you had no right calling yourself a world champion.

He speaks from experience. Back in October 1981, a young Mancini fought gallantly against the great Alexis Argüello for the WBC world lightweight title in what was his first world title shot, but was stopped in round fourteen. The fight was close at that point. Mancini had been narrowly ahead. 'If it's twelve rounds, I win the title,' Ray says. 'I was ahead on all three cards after twelve rounds. That's why I say this repeatedly: the true championship distance is fifteen rounds, not twelve. The history of boxing would be changed if it wasn't. Joe Louis would never have beaten Billy Conn. He was losing big after twelve. Rocky Marciano doesn't beat Joe Walcott. He was behind on all cards going into the thirteenth round. Ray Leonard doesn't beat Tommy Hearns. He's way behind going into the fourteenth round. You understand? The history of boxing would be completely changed. If it's over twelve rounds, I'm an undefeated champion.'

Let's take it further. Mancini would not only have beaten Argüello over twelve rounds in 1981, he'd have also regained his WBA title in June 1984, when Livingston Bramble, an unheralded challenger from St Kitts and Nevis, outlasted and stopped him in round fourteen. Again, Ray was leading on the cards at the time.

Then there's the other fourteenth-round stoppage on his record, a 1982 win against Korean Duk Koo Kim. Forget claiming and retaining world titles, if *that* fight had been scheduled for twelve rounds rather than fifteen, Kim, stopped in the fourteenth only to later lose his life, may have lived to fight another day. *Maybe*. 'I can't say that,' says Ray when I unfairly put the question to him. 'I really can't say that. Yeah, you can say if it was twelve rounds, he could still be alive, but maybe it would have been even more brutal because we only had to go twelve instead of fifteen. Maybe the twelve rounds would have been even more fast-paced.' Mancini shrugs, then shakes his head. He looks to the ground. 'You can't question that. Look, if the outcome was to be different, yes, I wish it had been a twelve-round fight. But we don't know that the outcome would have been different.'

Many, including the aforementioned *Express and Star*, have proposed the outcome of the fight between Mancini and Kim in 1982 was the reason behind boxing's various sanctioning bodies' decision to outlaw fifteen-round championship fights in 1987 and 1988. The World Boxing Association (WBA), World Boxing Council (WBC) and International Boxing Federation (IBF), the three major sanctioning bodies, all reduced their title fights from fifteen rounds to twelve rounds, thus shedding what they perceived were unnecessary dog rounds, but Mancini smiles when pinpointed as the reason for this change. 'They say that, but the last fifteen-round fight was 1988. That's six years after the Kim fight. That's a long time. If they were looking to make a change because of what happened with me and Kim, it was a long time coming. Ignore what they say. It was only ever a TV decision. The twelve-round fights work better for TV. You have more time for advertisements, you have more free time before and after fights. That's why the decision was made to go from fifteen rounds to twelve. It had nothing to do with injuries or anything medical. I know guys who worked for networks and they told me. I know the truth.'

DOG ROUNDS

The last fifteen-rounder sanctioned by the WBC was a heavyweight fight between Mike Tyson and Tyrell Biggs on 16 October 1987, while the last sanctioned by the WBA was the heavyweight fight between Evander Holyfield and Dwight Muhammad Qawi on 5 December 1987. The IBF, meanwhile, was the last to strip back to twelve rounds. They sanctioned a fifteen-round featherweight title fight between Jorge Páez and Calvin Grove on 4 August 1988, as well as a minimumweight title fight between Samuth Sithnaruepol and In-Kyu Hwang on 29 August. 'It ain't the same now,' Mancini sighs. 'Usually the first couple of rounds are the feeling-out rounds. They don't get down to business like we used to. It's a very different sport nowadays.'

No doubt there have been some ferocious twelve-rounders in the intervening years, but, in losing the fifteen-round championship distance – for reasons apparently owing to health and safety (or television scheduling) – so went a certain mindset and attitude. Nowadays, there's far more talk of hit and not getting hit, of minimising risk and of earning obscene amounts of money, all the while retaining one's faculties. Great, if you can achieve that, and irrefutably the sensible approach, but it's an option Mancini doesn't believe would have been viable for most back in his day. Fifteen rounders, he says, would have separated the businessmen from the boxers and the ones who really wanted, nay, *needed* to fight from the ones who were athletically gifted enough to make money from an ideology – a fight, a tear-up – to which they were actually opposed.

'I was never afraid of confrontation. It never meant anything to me. I liked that challenge – one man against another. I'm pitting myself against a gentleman who is physically, emotionally and spiritually different, yet we weigh the same and are both fighters. And one of us is getting carried out of there. That's the challenge. That I enjoy. People often say, "Were you ever scared?" I say, "Yeah, I was scared in every fight." But I wasn't scared of my opponent. It was more the unknown. If I got hit on the chin, I might get dropped or knocked out. How am I going to react? If I get clipped on the chin and get hurt, how am I going to respond? If I get dropped and get up, how will I respond? It's the fear of the unknown, not the opponent.'

Little was known of Duk Koo Kim, the Korean against whom Mancini defended his WBA world lightweight title on 13 November 1982. The youngest of five children, he was born in Goseong County, Gangwon Province, South Korea on 8 January 1959, and, at the time of fighting Mancini, possessed a professional boxing record of 17–1–1, having only once competed outside Korea. In terms of a style breakdown, an aggressive southpaw with toughness was about the sum of it, and Mancini was unsure of the fight for all those reasons. The unknown, the lefty element, the toughness. He was also further deterred upon hearing that back in Korea they described Kim as 'Little Mancini'. Fighting a mirror image of himself would, he thought, only lead to one thing: a headache.

'Poverty is my teacher,' Kim once wrote in his journal. It's a line that goes some way to explaining his character, his struggle, his hunger. This was a man who worked as a baker, welder and waiter to make ends meet and, when that failed, slept under a bridge subsisting on crackers as well as on the floor of a boxing gym. By the time he was in position for a title shot at Caesars Palace, however, for which he would be paid $20,000 to Mancini's $250,000, Duk Koo's fiancée, Lee Young-Mee, was pregnant with their first child and the need to provide had never been greater; the need to conquer Mancini and poverty had never been greater.

One journalist, Royce Feour of the *Las Vegas Review-Journal*, caught a priceless glimpse of the Korean's driven mindset when he went to interview him inside his Vegas hotel room during fight week and spotted a cryptic phrase scrawled on the bedside lampshade.

'What does that say?' Feour asked Kim's translator.

'Live or die,' he was told.

Kill-or-be-killed, to use the English colloquialism, the message was loud and clear. Kim hadn't arrived in Las Vegas to succumb to Mancini and simply roll over. He had every intention of winning the fight and would stop at nothing to get his hands on the belt.

The lampshade story never got back to Ray. He'd hear only of its poignancy in the aftermath. The tiny bit of insight he did receive, though, arrived backstage at Caesars Palace on the night of the fight when, through a paper-thin wall separating them, he heard Kim pounding his fists against the lockers in his changing room. The sound was accompanied by high-pitched wails, a war cry, and Ray knew there and then Kim hadn't come to lie down.

And so it proved. One southpaw, Kim, against a converted southpaw, Mancini, they were, as many suspected, soon to play conjoined twins at Caesars Palace's new ten thousand-seater outdoor arena, where Frank Sinatra, by now a huge fan of 'Boom Boom', sat ringside, and was joined by the likes of former three-weight world champion Henry Armstrong, Willie Stargell, who had led the Pittsburgh Pirates to two World Series victories, and showbiz stars Robert Goulet and Lou Rawls, as well as many others. Celebrity interest was high. It always was with Mancini. CBS showcased his story and his style, and most of America adored one or the other or both.

The importance of Kim's supporting role in the drama, meanwhile, was clear the moment he raced towards Mancini and hurled a wild left hand by way of formal introduction. From there, the whole thing escalated. People sat up in their seats, eyes on stalks, as both boxers looked to take the other out in the first round. Mancini worked weighty hooks, Kim fired his straight left hand with confident regularity, and it wasn't long before those who doubted the challenger's worth, his right to a number-one contender slot, were nodding their heads in approval. Three minutes down, one round in the bag, it was apparent Kim belonged.

It was apparent, also, that Mancini had his hands full. The Youngstown hero may have excelled in the second, sucking it up and matching Kim punch for punch, but, in round three, he watched Kim get clattered by a combination inside and then, rather than cower or seek refuge, bounce on the spot, raise his hands high above his head, and devilishly smile. It was an overt display of stoicism: live or die. Kim would not go down without a fight, and the punches Mancini had previously landed on others, with the intent to hurt, were not going to have the same effect on him. He simply wouldn't allow it.

Quickly, the mismatch became a war of attrition as both boxers stood close, locked in, head on shoulder, and pounded the other's torso, ribs and liver with hooks and uppercuts, as though throwing shots at a stationary heavy bag; if punching were allowed in a rugby scrum, this is surely what it would resemble. The key for Mancini was that his hands worked quicker on the inside, whereas Kim, a touch slower, was longer and more deliberate with his punching.

This often meant Ray would land two or three to Kim's one when the pair were engaged in the scrum. With distance created, however, as was the case in round six when Kim hurt Mancini with wide hooks and lunges, the fight took on an altogether different complexion. Now Kim was the one landing the cleaner, crisper and more damaging blows, as his left hand, thrown like he was pitching a baseball, connected over and over again.

'It was the only time I ever felt like quitting [in a fight],' says Mancini. 'My body was hurting so much in the middle of that fight. We were banging heads and he was hitting me with so many shots. My head was throbbing. The body wanted to shut down but the mind wouldn't let it. I just had to keep going. You have those thoughts but you dismiss them and move on.'

By round ten, it appeared Mancini had stumbled upon a breakthrough of sorts. He somehow tamed Kim, capitalising perhaps on his tiredness, and was able to keep him on the ropes and tee off on him with a number of quick punches to the head and body. Kim, for once, didn't respond or retaliate; whereas before he enthusiastically punched inside, now he was using such moments as an excuse to hold and buy time; he paused on the ropes for a moment; he tried to spin Mancini around; he took a deep breath.

But then, just as before, Kim, close to faltering, rallied strongly to end the round, making it appear as if his momentary surrender, whether on the ropes or in clinches, was simply a tactic used to see if Mancini would punch himself out.

'The pace they've set has been torrid,' said Gil Clancy, commentating for CBS, in round eleven. 'It's like a thirty-round fight.'

For his efforts, Kim was now effectively blind, both eyes shut, and Mancini, also swollen and unrecognisable, made another dent in him when he landed a right uppercut in the eleventh, one which dropped an off-balance Kim to his knee, a flash knockdown missed by referee Richard Green.

Nearing empty, Kim was grateful for the reprieve at the start of round twelve when some tape came loose on the inside of his right glove and Green told his corner to sort out the issue before recommencing the fight. The Koreans chewed up every second they could. They made it count. Mancini, meanwhile, sensing the delay benefited Kim, prowled just a few metres away from the challenger's corner, eager to get at him and resume the action.

He went one better in round thirteen, beginning the round just as Kim had begun round one: 'Boom Boom' raced to the centre of the ring and snatched at anything he could find, treating Kim like a human piñata, and used his superior physical strength to manoeuvre his foe around the ring. Kim, blind, hurt and now wobbling ever so slightly, seemed overwhelmed by it all.

And yet, seconds later, he was back. Back to punching and back to being a nuisance for Mancini and the thousands of Americans in attendance. 'We say fatigue has set in, and I really thought that, but he then changes my mind,' said Ray Leonard on commentary. Clancy nodded in agreement. 'I've seen guys get their second wind, but what about their fourth and fifth wind?' he said. Later that round, Kim was described by the broadcast team as the 'underrated Kim', a concession that they, like everyone else, had severely overlooked him.

As Ray Mancini sat on his stool before round fourteen, having watched his cornermen depart the ring, he received his gum shield in his mouth and then crossed his chest and kissed his right glove. It wasn't supposed to have been this hard, he thought. But here we are. One last push. The champion then rose from his stool, the bell sounded and Kim repeated his trick from the first round – darting recklessly into the fire – only this time Mancini was wise to the move. He stepped around the onrushing challenger and landed two short hooks inside, both of which hurt Kim, who staggered and then froze momentarily. Mancini, senses still sharp so late in the fight, pounced in an instant. He followed with further punches, the most notable of which was a final straight right hand that pierced Kim's porous guard and sent him flying to the canvas, flat on his back, as if stood too near an explosion. It was, by definition, a finishing shot. It couldn't have been cleaner, truer or more emphatic.

Even so, Kim, during the ensuing count, somehow moved on to his side and got up to his knees. He tried to continue. Boy, did he try. A right glove pawed at the bottom rope, before finally connecting and grabbing it, and his left glove did the same with the rope second from bottom. Then, with his left hanging on for dear life, he used all remaining drops of energy to pull himself upright with every intention of carrying on. As far as acts of bravery go, it was perhaps his finest moment.

Referee Green, though, could see Kim was in no fit state to fight. He took control and ended the struggle.

'If that ending didn't happen, it would be one of those great fights you'd see on *ESPN Classic* all the time,' says Mancini. 'But, because Kim passed, it was never viewed like that. It changed the context of the fight.'

Moments after attempting to rise with the aid of ring ropes, Kim, averaging four breaths a minute, collapsed into a coma and was rushed to Desert Springs Hospital, where they discovered he had a subdural haematoma on the right side of his brain and that most of the blood had settled in the parietal lobe. The neurosurgeon, Dr Lonnie Hammargren, said the haemorrhage was relatively fresh and that the trauma may have even been the result of a single blow – the last. He also said Kim had very little chance of making it.

He was right. Twenty-three-year-old Duk Koo Kim, a number-one contender who melted the hearts of a Vegas crowd and showed an inordinate amount of potential on his biggest night, died four days after challenging Ray Mancini for the WBA world lightweight title. The date was 17 November 1982.

'I wanted to go to the funeral but decided not to,' says Ray. 'It has been reported that I attended, but I didn't. And it's a shame. I wanted to go and felt an obligation to do so. But a good friend of mine, a Korean, my mother and sister's karate teacher, contacted a friend of his in Korea to gauge the climate around that time and they said it would not be good for me to go. They would extend my condolences to his family and to the government instead.'

Kim was laid to rest in Kojin Village Cemetery, Gangwon-do, South Korea, while Mancini, a man who would now forever be associated with the fallen Korean, slipped into a slow, steady and serious depression. Righteous reasons a thing of the past, Ray, once the golden boy of CBS television and a man with countless endorsements in the pipeline, was now something of a pariah. Nobody knew quite what to say. Was he a boxer or a murderer? Was boxing itself a sport or a crime? Ray himself wasn't even sure any more. 'The perception of me changed a lot in the eyes of the public,' he says, thirty-three years later. 'I went from a guy who represented everything good about boxing – winning a world title for my father – to a guy who was the poster boy for all that was bad about boxing. And, just as winning the world title changes you, *that* also changes you. My Christian faith is the only thing that carried me through. If not, I might have taken the bridge, put the gun in my mouth, drank the bottle, taken the pills. If you're weak-minded, that's what happens. But, because of my faith and my mental strength, I was able to get through it.'

Eager to expunge the Kim tragedy from his mind, Mancini agreed to return to the ring just three months later, signing to fight England's George Feeney in Italy the following February. A non-title affair, belt not up for grabs, Mancini intended to use the ten rounds to test himself out, see how he felt, eradicate any bad thoughts and more or less go through the motions.

'I had to decide whether I was mentally and emotionally prepared to get back in there,' he says. 'You can't fight scared. Plus, my style wouldn't allow it. If I was going to try and carry on with my style but not be emotionally prepared to go where I used to go, I was going to get hurt. I'd become a danger to myself. I had to be fully committed and fully convinced it was the right decision. The problem I had was that my righteous reasons for boxing had now gone. That Kim fight made me fall out of love with the sport. At that point, boxing strictly became a business to me.'

There were bigger problems afoot. In a turn of events that only added depth to the tragedy, Kim's mother, Yang Sun Nyo, had had enough of the grieving, the family infighting and the emptiness in her heart and decided to take her own life. 'I was preparing for the Feeney fight when I heard the news of his mother's suicide,' recalls Ray. 'I was thinking, what's next? The European press were relentless. The press in general jumped on that and whupped my ass. I understood they had a job to do but the way they reported it was brutal. It took its toll on me. I went through it all over again.'

Mancini was no stranger to tragedy. In fact, a year before the death of Kim, Ray had to come to terms with losing his older brother, Lenny Jr, who died from a gunshot wound administered by his seventeen-year-old girlfriend, Diana Kirkwood, on 14 February 1981. She claimed she accidentally discharged the gun while he was showing her how to use it, and later pleaded guilty to negligent homicide, a misdemeanour, and was remanded to the custody of the Ohio Youth Commission. Ray's brother was dead, though, robbed of the chance of ever seeing him lift the world lightweight championship, and anger, of which there was plenty, had to somehow be displaced by an even greater appetite to succeed and illuminate the Mancini name. It was the only way.

Unfairly, by the time he faced Feeney, the Mancini name had other connotations. Gone was the father–son association and the idea that this sweet boy from Youngstown had overcome the odds, as well as tragedy, to win the world lightweight championship. That had been replaced by an altogether darker image, one of Mancini celebrating his win over Kim oblivious to the fact his Korean opponent would soon slip into a coma and die four days later. Unwarranted, it nevertheless stuck. Even worse, it followed him to Italy, where he soon discovered he was the key protagonist in an international news story and that the European press were just as unforgiving as those he had encountered back in the United States. They harangued him. They misquoted him. Mancini soon became sick of them. He wanted the fight finished and he wanted to go home.

'The Feeney fight was the only time I got in the ring and didn't care whether I won or lost,' he says. 'Feeney never had a better chance to beat me than that night. I was ripe for the taking. My mind was somewhere else. It wasn't an impressive fight. I wasn't the same. I was emotionally and mentally drained. I had nothing. I'm sure when I landed a few times on George Feeney, he'd have been thinking, boy, is *this* the world champion? Is this all he's got? That's all I had that day. I just wanted it all to be over.'

Mancini claimed a close decision, by scores of 98–96, 98–96 and 98–95, after ten completed rounds. For a world champion supposedly on the rise, though, it was a dud.

Later that year, in July 1983, two further developments in the Kim tragedy brought it all back to Mancini. First off, the referee that night, Richard Green, forty-six, died from a self-inflicted gunshot wound to the head inside his Las Vegas home, and then, secondly, Kim's fiancée, Lee Young-Mee, gave birth to a boy, Kim Chi-Wan, who'd grow up to become a dentist and, in 2011, would, alongside his mother, meet Mancini as part of *The Good Son* documentary.

'Boom Boom' still tried to forget. He wouldn't watch the fight or even talk about it for a number of years. It was too raw, too fresh, too painful. In reality, it wasn't until his daughter, Carmenina, came home from school one day with a question that he finally decided to sit down and revisit the very thing that had haunted him through much of the eighties. Crying Carmenina, eight years of age, told her father that a boy at basketball practice had accused him of ending another man's life.

'Popi, Popi, he called you a murderer,' she said.

'Popi's not a murderer,' he answered. 'Why do you say that?'

'He said, "Your dad killed someone in a boxing ring."'

Ray shook his head.

'Is it true, Popi?'

Ray knew there'd come a time when he'd have to open up to his daughter. He just didn't know when. 'I sat her down, I explained it to her and then I put on the fight,' he recalls. 'I sat and watched it with her from beginning to end. At the end of the fight she turned to me and said, "Popi, that's just something that happened." I said, "Yes. Now you understand."'

Mancini's final professional fight took place in April 1992, three years after a loss to Héctor Camacho, and was against Greg Haugen for the lightly regarded NABF (North American Boxing Federation) light-welterweight title. Haugen was a former IBF world lightweight champion and had also lost his WBO world light-welterweight title to Camacho two fights before facing Mancini. Ray, on the other hand, had just been doing an off-Broadway play in New York when he got the call to fight again.

'Whenever I'm asked by people about retirement, I always say I retired in 1985, not 1992,' he says. 'Coming back for one fight in four years, then taking another fight three years later, doesn't constitute an active fighter. Camacho was personal. I thought I was young enough to do it. I was twenty-eight. It wasn't like I was coming back to fight Julio César Chávez. I knew I could handle Camacho. Haugen was the same. When they offered it to me, I thought, tough guy, stands in front of you, can't punch much, takes a good ass-kicking, the type of guy I love to fight. That was pure ego. I wasn't being physically challenged with the acting and I wanted to see if I could still compete like a world-class athlete.'

At first, the signs were good. Mancini trained like a world-class athlete, he broke all his old records and he seemed as good as new. There was no suggestion he'd slowed or that his love for the game had fizzled out. If anything, his body convinced his mind it was a good idea.

But, three months before he began his camp in February, his son, Leonardo, was born and Ray, now in the throes of training, couldn't shake the guilt he felt when leaving him. It was there with him whenever he ran, whenever he sparred or whenever he simply sat and ate. Most days he'd take a nap from ten o'clock to two o'clock, get up, watch television, start to get ready and then make his way to the gym for four. At three o'clock, though, while in the process of getting dressed, Ray would habitually start to break down and cry, and the reason for this was Eric Clapton's 'Tears from Heaven', a song written about the pain and loss Clapton felt following the death of his young son, Conor, which came on the radio every day at three seemingly for no other reason than to test Mancini. Each time he failed. 'I'd be bawling like a baby,' Ray says. 'I couldn't control it. I missed my children. I said to myself, "This ain't good." I was beaten before I got in the ring. I knew I couldn't fight any more.'

On the night of the Haugen fight, having dragged himself through the hardest training camp of his career, Mancini finally came clean. Sitting in one of the Reno-Sparks Convention Center changing rooms, he leaned towards his trainer, Chuck Fagan, and said, 'Chuck, I don't want to be here. I don't want to do this.'

Chuck frowned. 'Well,' he said, 'it's a hell of a time to tell me, ain't it?'

While he may have trained like a world-class fighter, Mancini was no longer able to think or perform like one. Immense pride got him to the ring against Haugen, but he was stopped in seven rounds, the first and only stoppage loss of his career, and never contemplated fighting again.

'Before fights I'd always be of the mindset that one of us was getting carried out of there – either him or me,' he says. 'I was fearless. But that night it was more like, "Please God, don't let me get hurt. My babies need me." Napoleon said – and you didn't know I could quote Napoleon, did you? – that after the age of thirty a man's spirit is not made for war. He meant your values change, your ideology changes, *everything* changes. The only good thing about that Haugen fight was that I resolved it. There were no longer any what-ifs.'

Some things were left unresolved, mind. Duk Koo Kim for one. Discussing it privately with family members and his priest, Father Tim O'Neill, went some way to healing open wounds, but Mancini refused to talk about the incident publicly until ESPN approached him about doing a documentary to commemorate its twenty-fifth anniversary. The documentary was to be called *Triumph and Tragedy*, and they wanted Ray's involvement. 'No way,' he initially said, before ESPN made it clear they were going to persevere with the project with or without his assistance. 'Well, in that case, count me in,' he said, U-turn complete. Years later, he explains, 'If they had to do it, I wasn't going to have anyone else tell the story. I wanted it in my own words.'

That was only the first stumbling block. Next, ESPN sought permission to retrieve footage of the lost fight, hidden from the public for twenty-five years, from its promoter Bob Arum. Mancini made the all-important call. 'Look, Bob, I appreciate you protecting me all these years, and that you stuck to your word, but they can't do a piece on it without the viewers seeing the fight,' he said. 'Without seeing the fight, people will not understand the full scope of it. They'll think I just went out there and walked through this guy and beat him up. They'll think it was a mismatch and that I overwhelmed him. They won't appreciate that the fight was give-and-take and that he was a formidable opponent. We can talk about it as much as we want, but nothing convinces quite like moving images. They need to see it for themselves.'

Arum released the footage on Mancini's request, the documentary was made and the hope was that it would clear up some of the mystery, dispel some of the rumours and allow viewers to watch the horror for themselves before making up their own minds. Moreover, Mancini, finally, could speak about something he'd avoided for over two decades. It was, in essence, a forty-five-minute confession.

'It's a fact of life, a part of life,' he says now. 'A friend of mine said, "Raymond, why did all these things happen to you?" I said, "Why *not* me? Why should I be exempt? What makes me so damn special?" I'm a firm believer that the good Lord puts things in our life to grow our faith and to develop as people and to get stronger. I've dealt with things in my life and it has only made me lean on Him more. In that respect, I appreciate everything in my life. The good and the bad. I don't always think, why did it happen? The things I've gone through have helped me become the man I am today. Everything in life changes you. Tao, the Chinese philosophy, says everything changes; the leaves on the trees, blades of grass, the birds in the air. All things change. If you resist change, you open yourself up for heartache and pain. That's very deep. It means a lot to me. I can't imagine being one of those people who doesn't have faith. I can't imagine what a lonely existence it is to go through life thinking that once you're dead they put you in a black box and that's it. Man, we're not cereal boxes. We don't have expiration dates. We need to believe that there's more to this life. I look forward to the next life, I really do, but I'm going to keep enjoying this one for as long as I've got.'

While attending the 2002 premiere of *Champion*, a Korean film based on the life of Duk Koo Kim, Mancini was told of an Asian philosophy that, he felt, explained why the Korean people believe the spirit of Kim now continues to flow through him. A sentiment in line with his own set of beliefs, he stopped for a moment to take it all in, then responded in kind by saying Duk Koo Kim was never far from his mind and that he hoped they'd one day be reunited. 'There are a few up there waiting for me,' he said.

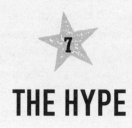

THE HYPE

Grudge match, they say. Bad blood, no love lost, they say. Fights sell better that way. Stir it up. Push buttons. Stoke the fire. Light the blue touchpaper. It all helps at the box office. It makes us all money. The fighters get it, too. They'll say some churlish things about each other, act like they mean it and then add the all-important disclaimer either just before or just after the fight: nothing personal, just business.

Nick Blackwell and Chris Eubank Jr were no different. Their not-so-unique brand of locally sourced beef started the moment they agreed to fight one another for the British middleweight title. Once signed, Blackwell accused his challenger of ducking him on three prior occasions and boasted of getting the better of him once upon a time in sparring, while Eubank Jr, in retaliation, labelled the British champion bland and said he was doing the belt a disservice.

Yada, yada, for weeks it rolled on like this, as I poked and prodded both, engaged them in a game of he-said-she-said, and then ducked for cover whenever I sensed one of them was summoning a hearty dose of phlegm to gob the other way. They were, for all intents and purposes, warring neighbours, slinging mud over a separating fence, and I, the press officer, was meddling Maureen from three doors down discreetly slipping hate mail and dog faeces through their letterboxes. I felt no way about it, either. It was all part of the game.

'It's never personal, always business,' explained Eubank Jr. 'I'm fighting him not because I don't like him but because he has a title I want. It doesn't matter whether he likes me or hates me. And that goes for everyone who is watching the fight as well. You can love me or loathe me, but so long as you're watching, I'm happy.'

On this point, Blackwell agreed. 'I never take a fight personally,' he said. 'I don't particularly like him or his attitude, but I don't take any of his nonsense personally. I just don't agree with the way he goes about things. Hate is a strong word and I don't know enough about the real Chris Eubank Jr to say I hate him. All I have got to go on is a persona he and his father have created. He's a fake. He's trying to be someone he's not. He could actually be a nice kid if he cut the apron strings and was himself a bit more, but he's told what to say by his father and he's always in performance mode. There's nothing real about him.'

There it is, that animosity bubbling beneath the surface, acting as ammunition. It was all I needed. They claimed it wasn't personal, but I wanted to make it personal. It was my job, as press officer, to make them hate each other. It was, history said, the simplest and cheapest way to sell a fight.

'It's laughable for him to say I've been avoiding him,' said Eubank Jr. 'He's a boring guy. He has to say something to try and get some attention but his stories about me avoiding him are fantasy. It's not good for boxing if he's the British champion. They need someone who is really going to fly the flag and inspire and excite people. I'm going to take the belts from him and make the British public proud.'

Okay, Blackwell, now your turn.

'It's all nonsense. If we're talking about doing the British title a disservice, how could anybody possibly look up to Chris Eubank Jr? He's the furthest thing from a role model you can get. People in boxing never have anything good to say about him. You never hear someone say, "Oh, yeah, he's a decent guy." If some young kid was getting into boxing and the first boxer they came across was Chris Eubank Jr, they'd be put off the sport for life. They'd think every boxer was as arrogant, unlikeable and big-headed as him. If he was to ever get lucky enough to win a British title, and I don't think he ever will, it will be a sad day.'

It started to get personal, even if they said it wouldn't. And, as the hate increased, so did the grandstanding.

'I'll capitalise on Blackwell's weak defence,' said Eubank Jr. 'I've watched his last few fights and nothing I've seen impresses or worries me. He's a British-level fighter and I'm world-level. The public will see the difference once we step in the ring. Whether he quits, gets stopped or gets knocked out, he's not making it to the final bell. If he wants to go in there and be the big I am, Mr Big Man, who's not scared of Chris Eubank Jr, then he will get knocked out.'

'Let him think he's the bigger puncher,' answered Blackwell. 'When he gets in there with me and is breathing out his arse and getting hit flush, he'll realise I hit a lot harder than my record might suggest. He won't want to be taking it on the chin from me in ten-ounce gloves. No chance.'

Hate also fuelled the meeting of Chris Eubank and Michael Watson at White Hart Lane on 21 September 1991. I say hate, that's probably a tad strong – in both instances – but there's certainly a professional, organised (business not personal) hate that exists between boxers, a necessary hate, and it is usually sparked by competition or a personality clash or simply the primeval notion that one man is about to fight another. It takes a strong character not to get caught up in all that and therefore not become emotionally invested.

In terms of Eubank and Watson, their animosity stemmed from competition. More accurately, it was a product of Watson's steadfast belief that he'd been robbed of victory in their first encounter, held three months earlier at Earl's Court, and that Eubank was handed a majority decision victory on account of his greater star power. Eubank, of course, strongly refuted this claim. It was a close fight, he agreed, but the three ringside judges voted in his favour. Enough said. Case closed. The majority of those who watched, it should be noted, tended to side with Watson. But, whatever. The only way to settle the squabble was to do it all over again and clear up the ambiguity. Do it bigger next time, sell it harder, make more money. The first fight at Earl's Court, with a WBO world middleweight title on the line, was just that – a fight. The rematch, however, was by now a grudge match big enough in scope to play out in front of over 20,000 people at a football stadium. You had Eubank on one side, Watson on the other. Their distinct roles were clear. The storyline was in place. Britain, a nation invested in the drama, wanted to see them beat each other up in the name of some sort of conclusion.

'He has pushed boxing down to the gutter,' said Watson

of Eubank. 'You've got the greats like Marvin Hagler and "Sugar" Ray Leonard putting boxing on the map, and this man has totally torn boxing apart. It really makes me feel bad. I won the last fight, but getting Chris Eubank out of my system, beating Chris Eubank, is my first priority. Becoming world champion is secondary.'

'I have a lot of contempt for this man, for his frame of mind,' Eubank responded. 'His point of view is weak. This is what I see and detect from his personality. I don't like him, I don't dislike him. He's not even there. I don't regard him as anything. Who is he? I don't know who this man is. He's an obstacle that is going to be in front of me on the twenty-first of September and he's an obstacle I must pass. Other than that, he doesn't exist.'

Sound familiar? Things heated up further when the pair met at a press conference to officially announce their WBO world super-middleweight title fight at White Hart Lane. Now face to face, their true feelings showed; Eubank, especially, was unable to hold back, so wounded was he by the accusation that he'd received a gift decision following their fight in June.

'You make me sick,' he told Watson across the top table. 'You're pitiful. You lost the fight.'

'You're kidding yourself,' replied Watson.

'You think so?'

'I *know* so.'

'Let me explain something. Before the fight, I said I wouldn't begrudge you the win. You've begrudged me the win. I won the fight. Accept that and stop whinging like a child. You're going on like you're some kind of big shot, but if I got up and walked out this room, you'd be left starving. Be quiet.'

'Ask these people here who is carrying on like the big shot,' said Watson, grinning, pointing to the press.

'I'm just talking. I'm making a statement. If I was to get up and walk out this room...'

'Relax, calm down.'

'There's no calming down. This guy's an idiot, man. You're a complete and utter idiot, that's what you are. Nah, I'm done with this press conference, man. Let me go or I'm going to whack his ears off.'

'Bye, Chris.'

It was unmistakeably Eubank – who else could get away with labelling their opponent a 'complete and utter idiot' and threatening to 'whack his ears off' days before a fight? – but he was no longer playing a part or acting up. He was serious. He seemed uncharacteristically vexed and emotional. Watson, the designated 'People's Champion', was cooler, calmer and more popular than he was. He had the support of the nation on his side. He was good, safe, wholesome. He represented justice. And Chris Eubank, the competitor, hated – yes, *hated* – that.

On the eve of his third British title defence, Nick Blackwell sits with friends in the bar of Wembley's Holiday Inn – which, for one night only, masquerades as a man cave in Trowbridge – and, while those around him sink pints of beer and Guinness, he's content to slowly sip from a cup of coffee and a bottle of water. He listens to his trainer, Gary Lockett, tell jokes and do impressions, and laughs as freely as he would on any other evening, for these are his people, this is his moment.

At one point Nick is handed a brown package containing the black and gold robe he'll wear en route to the ring the following night. The package is immediately ripped open and the robe held aloft for all to see. 'You've changed,' one of his friends wisecracks. 'Look at it. All sparkly and stuff.'

Nick smiles. 'I can't wait to smash him in the face with a right hand,' he says.

He is getting agitated and impatient, and the presence of the robe brings it all back. It acts as a reminder that a fight is now just twenty-four hours away. Tick-tock, tick-tock. All of a sudden Lockett's impersonations dry up, his friends drink up, and Nick finishes his coffee, signals he is turning in for the night, then leaves on his own. We shake hands and I wonder how well he'll sleep.

The next morning, as I queue for breakfast, Nick shimmies towards me, throws a playful combination of punches at my stomach, and then stops to listen to the very question which had been bothering me. 'How did you sleep?' I say.

The ever-present smile on his face stretches wider. 'Like a baby,' he replies.

A couple of hours later I am hidden away in one of the offices of Wembley Arena with the Hennessy Sports event manager, Lee Squirrell, handling two pairs of ten-ounce boxing gloves wrapped in plastic bags. One pair is branded Grant, the other Winning. The Grant ones will eventually find their way on to the fists of Nick Blackwell and the Winning ones will be worn by Chris Eubank Jr. Together, we marvel at the differences in the gloves. Both weigh the same (only the distribution of weight differs from brand to brand), but the Winning gloves, we agree, are noticeably larger than the Grant ones, with plenty more padding around the knuckle, whereas the Grant gloves carry their weight in the wrist area. 'I know which ones I'd rather be getting hit in the face with,' says Lee. He means the Winning gloves. Eubank

Jr's gloves. The bigger ones. The seemingly safer ones. And I am in total agreement.

Our next job as promoters of the event is to sort out payment slips and cash for all the boxers, managers, officials and doctors who will later appear in this very office and await payment from Squirrell. This is a laborious, mind-numbing task, which consists of counting endless twenty-pound notes, writing names on invoices and sealing envelopes, but remains insightful nonetheless. How else is one ever to know how much a judge or referee gets paid on fight night? The doctors, for example, will tonight pocket between five hundred and seven hundred pounds each. 'Nice work if you can get it,' I say.

'Yeah, not bad for just sitting around and watching fights for a few hours,' says Lee.

'Whenever you're a mandatory requirement, you can effectively name your price, I guess.'

'Exactly. But when you think about how often they're actually needed or used...'

The fight between Blackwell and Eubank Jr is to be screened from 9:40p.m. on Channel 5 and the broadcasters hope, given the bad blood between the pair and the power of the Eubank brand, they might eclipse the 3.2 million viewers who tuned in to watch the British heavyweight title fight between Tyson Fury and Dereck Chisora in 2011. Or at least get close. What Channel 5 also hope for are enough competitive fights to fill a time slot spanning over two hours. This is made abundantly clear the moment Mark Sharman, Channel 5's boxing producer, enters our office in a tizzy and somehow condenses two human beings with beating hearts, about to put their lives on the line for our entertainment, into cold, hard statistics.

THE HYPE

'I'm really worried this one might go short,' he says, pacing the room. 'Eubank looked impressive at the weigh-in, didn't he? Powerful. Explosive.'

'Don't worry,' I say. 'It won't go short. Nick is too tough and I don't believe Eubank hits hard enough for it to go short.'

'I've just got a feeling.'

'Even if Eubank does win, it will go long. You'll get what you want.'

'I'm hoping for at least eight rounds.'

'Yeah, you'll get that.'

Television will get that. You will get that. I will get that. We will all get that. But at what price?

Like it matters. None of us are paying. Not him, not me, not you. We just sit back and wait and speculate and rub our hands together and rub our bellies and hope we get the kind of violence that leaves us sufficiently nourished. On fight day, while bored in the office, I will even take to Twitter to tweet the following: *Got a feeling Blackwell vs. Eubank Jr is going to be one of those fights that's almost hard to watch. It will be carnage. Can't wait.*

It reads like I'm placing an order. I mean every word of it.

THE MASOCHIST I

Gabriel Ruelas is ready to die. He was ready to die years ago. He even sometimes dreams of dying – mostly in car wrecks and plane crashes, ironically never in the boxing ring – and bears a tattoo of a man shaking hands with a skeleton on his arm. When the end nears, it will come as no surprise. He's gearing up for it, every additional day an inconvenience, and the sense of relief he'll feel when finally, properly greeting death is one of the few things that keeps him going nowadays; this despite the fact he's still only forty-five years of age, lives a presumably happy life in Los Angeles, California and has two sons, Diego, twenty-one, and Rodrigo, seventeen, with his wife, Leslie.

'The doctors say my mind is in the category of sixty-five years old and over,' explains the bespectacled Ruelas at home, flecks of grey in his otherwise jet-black, spiky hair. 'I have a medical card that allows me to go certain places. It's like being disabled. I keep thinking, when am I going to go? I always dreamed of dying young and that hasn't changed. I've been fascinated by death since I was a kid.'

The other day, Gabriel was asked by Leslie, who understandably cannot abide this obsession with death, to list his hobbies in an attempt to steer him away from the subject of his own mortality and direct his thoughts towards somewhat healthier pursuits. But, try as he might, the former WBC world super-featherweight champion came up blank. His list was depressingly slight. By way of an apology, he explained to Leslie that he had achieved and received all he had ever wanted from life – a world title, two sons, a 'white woman who now speaks Spanish' – and to wish for anything more would amount to pure greed on his part. Still, on the list of hobbies were reading newspapers – the *Los Angeles Times* and *La Opinión*, in particular – scouring Facebook, though he admits computers confuse him, and also staying active, though he's no longer able to run the way he did during his heyday through fear of getting lost. When Gabe runs, he runs far. So far he sometimes disappears. It has happened. Leslie has lost him on more than one occasion. It has got so bad now, in fact, that when Gabe leaves the house, which isn't too often these days, there's a need for constant communication with his wife, who ensures he has his phone with him in his pocket at all times. Without it, he's prone to forgetting the objective of his trip.

'It's scary,' he says. 'A few times I have gone out the house to do something and I've forgotten *everything*. I forget where I am, what I'm doing and where I'm supposed to be going. Life is hard for me now. It's better to be dead, I think, than scared all the time. I don't want people to feel sorry for me. I try to act normal with the people around me – family, friends – but I really don't feel normal. I'm a very good liar. I fool a lot of them. Sometimes I just want to leave this place because I don't want to be a burden. Where I come from [La Yerbabuena, Jalisco, Mexico, a remote place up in the mountains, four hours from Guadalajara, population one hundred, where Gabe lived with his father, Rafael, his mother, Maria, as well as a number of siblings], we didn't have hospitals, we didn't have homes where people are taken care of. I wouldn't want my family to be taking care of me. I'd rather live somewhere by myself. We still have a place in the ranch in Mexico. I could live out the rest of my days there. I'd rather live that way. People there just live a normal life. Nobody knows anything. You live like an animal, but a happy animal. You don't have to deal with the stress of everyday life in Los Angeles.'

Midway through our interview, Ruelas gets up from his chair in a kind of blind panic, and realises he has bought two identical copies of the Spanish paper *La Opinión*. There's your stress. Unintentional, it's something he does from time to time; The *Los Angeles Times*, his other favourite paper, gets delivered to his door every morning, but fetching his Spanish paper requires him leaving his home and finding the nearest vending machine, which often causes confusion as Gabe forgets whether he has or hasn't already bought the newspaper that day. 'I do my best,' he says. 'Before I get it out of the machine, I look at the paper and I'm like, "Okay, does it look familiar? Does it look like something I've seen before?" I shake my head and say, "No, it doesn't look familiar."

'Sure enough, though, when I get home, I see the paper already in the house. Every time I buy two papers I know it's a sign my memory is getting worse.'

'Is the loss of memory boxing-related?' I ask, presuming a fifteen-year professional boxing career is to blame.

'Not at all,' he says. 'Well, maybe a little part of it is due to boxing, but most of it is because of the trauma I suffered in 1995. It's all the emotional and psychological stuff I went through after Jimmy Garcia.'

Back in 1995, Ruelas knew little about his next world title challenger, only that he came from Colombia, was likely to be a soft touch and that he deserved the kind of hurting saved for opponents he truly disliked. That was the general assessment of Jimmy Garcia once Ruelas heard the mulleted South American had upset his wife with a comment directed her way around the Caesars Palace pool the day before their May fight in Las Vegas. He suspected Garcia would be overmatched and out of his depth beforehand, but now he *really* wanted to prove the point. Now he wanted to punish Garcia for disrespecting his girl.

Ruelas can't recall what Garcia was alleged to have said to Leslie, and concedes it may have simply been a look or a gesture, but, whatever it was, it stuck with him. It stuck with him that day and it stuck with him the next day, too, when scheduled to face Garcia over twelve rounds in defence of his WBC world super-featherweight title. A switch had been flicked in Gabe and Leslie, knowing how her husband could get when wound up, was quick to apologise for telling him what Garcia had said. She didn't like seeing the impact it had on her husband. He was enraged. All focus was lost. He was back to street-fightin' Gabe Ruelas. 'I'm going to make him pay,' he promised her. 'The next time I see him, he's going to get it.'

Gabe wished the fight was to take place on Friday night, not Saturday night. He shadowboxed with a purpose in his hotel room on the eve of battle, imagining Garcia on the end of his punches, and told himself, over and over again, that it was a mismatch, a joke fight, and that Garcia, boxing outside his native Colombia for only the fourth time, would be found woefully out of his depth. 'I didn't know much about Jimmy, but I knew he had just lost to Genaro Hernández,' recalls Gabe. 'I thought, if this guy lost to Genaro Hernández, why the hell am I fighting him? Is he a leftover for me or something? Anyhow, I had to do what I had to do and he was who they wanted me to fight.'

A professional boxer since July 1988, Jimmy Garcia was about to compete in his fortieth pro fight against Ruelas. During this time, he had boxed twice in Panama, once in Mexico, and the rest of his fights had taken place in Colombia. There were four defeats on his record; three nondescript points losses; one to Genaro Hernández in a WBA world super-featherweight title fight. That shot at Hernández's belt came six months before his fight with Ruelas and Garcia lost near enough every round and was on the receiving end of lopsided scorecards which read 120–107, 119–109 and 117–109. His reward? Another chance.

When Gabe and Jimmy eventually took to the ring outside at Caesars Palace, the same spot where Ray Mancini tragically felled Duk Koo Kim thirteen years earlier, it was still light. The stands were slowly filling in anticipation of the main event (which featured Gabe's younger brother, Rafael, challenging Oscar De La Hoya for his IBF and WBO world lightweight titles), and most who'd bothered to leave the casinos viewed gung-ho Gabe as an ideal appetiser. He was, for a time, as good a Roberto Durán impersonator as there'd ever been. Visually, his mop of black hair and eyes, which seemed to darken the closer he got to the first bell, were straight from the 'Hands of Stone' textbook, while tics such as head-bobbing, foot-shuffling and an incessant pursuit of the knockout could only have been developed from studying the great Panamanian. For the early birds in attendance, he was a wonderful tribute act, and never had anyone made Gabriel Ruelas look more like Roberto Durán than Jimmy Garcia on 6 May 1995. Quick out of the blocks, Gabe stalked Jimmy from the off, channelling Durán, and slung haphazard left hooks his way and hurried to deliver follow-up blows, so eager was he to finish the fight early and settle into his seat for the main event. The crowd, similarly impatient, acted in kind – oohing and aahing his every attempt – and, within seconds of the opening round unfolding, it seemed only a matter of time before poor Jimmy Garcia was put out of his misery, as wild left hooks that would normally be blocked, parried or evaded altogether, such was their directness, clattered into his face and brought his head up, the tail of his mullet flying in the wind.

'I was hitting him very freely, which surprised me,' recalls Gabe. 'I didn't see him act like he was hurt by many of them, though. Normally I'd hit opponents with the same shots and they'd be badly hurt. These were *clean* shots. I just thought, man, this guy can take a punch. Sometimes you hit someone and you don't see any reaction and it can be disheartening. You know you're hitting him hard but you don't see anything. I was, like, damn, what's up with this guy? I saw nothing on his face. He had no expression. I didn't know what he was thinking.'

All Jimmy offered in response was a negative, tepid jab, which he used to almost measure the distance between himself and Ruelas rather than hurt the champion. He touched him to the head with this punch, a term used lightly, and then touched him to the body with awkward hooks. Only ever touches, mind. 'Jimmy doesn't seem to have any power whatsoever,' said HBO commentator and world super-middleweight champion Roy Jones Jr, watching from ringside. Hip to this, Gabe would occasionally wait for Garcia to get busy with his jab, which he did when given space, and then time it so he exploded over the top of it with a right hand of his own, much to the delight of the watching crowd. It was a cruel spectacle, not far off bear-baiting. 'This guy just takes shot after shot after shot,' added Jones Jr.

Ruelas sat down in his corner after two rounds and Joe Goossen, his curmudgeonly trainer, looked more miserable than usual in a pristine white tracksuit. His boy was winning, and winning well, but it could apparently be made even easier if he'd just goddamn listen to him. 'There's no reason to give him three-, four- or five-second intervals in between punches,' he said. 'It's constant pressure on this guy. He hasn't done one offensive thing to you. There's no reason to even think he's going to do something. Keep your hands up and walk through this guy. But you've got to do it with some style. You can't just keep winging them. I want you to get to the body.'

In Garcia's corner, meanwhile, the challenger was instructed by his brother, Manuel Jr, to simply throw three punches at a time, use his legs and walk away; trade vernacular for 'run for your life'.

With thirty seconds to go in round three, Ruelas finally appeared to hurt Garcia – *properly* hurt him – as he cracked the point of his chin with two left hooks, the second of which made Garcia's eyes roll in his head and his knees buckle. For lesser men, it would have proved to be a knockout shot, that much was certain. But Garcia, if nothing else, possessed a kind of superhuman tolerance to pain, an almost unfortunate level of durability, and this allowed him to move, spoil and eventually see out the round.

'He can't hurt you,' Goossen told Ruelas before round four. In many ways, that was the saddest element of all. Garcia, drained from losing thirty-two pounds in a month, was ostensibly battling an armed assassin with a spud gun. There was nothing on his pokes and prods and his body, lacking muscle definition and very narrow, was easily shoved around by Ruelas whenever the champion felt like putting him in the right position for crippling hooks and uppercuts. 'You've got to get the liver,' Goossen continued. 'How many times have I got to tell you? You're winning every round but you could be putting a hurtin' on this guy to the left side.'

Ruelas began the sixth with a crazy lead left uppercut, which again landed clean, but then settled down a little. His work-rate dropped. Not exactly tired, he nevertheless seemed bored of abusing Garcia. He'd hit him by now with every punch in the book – the jab, the cross, the hook, countless uppercuts and savage digs to the body, too – and was perhaps now wondering, what else can I do? Added to that there was nothing coming back to keep him on his toes, keep him sharp, keep him awake, keep him interested.

'Jimmy can take everything,' said Jones Jr. 'I don't care what you hit him with. He can take it.'

'One of the great mysteries of the sport, Roy, is why some fighters have a beard [chin] and some don't,' added HBO's Jim Lampley.

'Indeed. I don't know whether I have a beard or not. And I don't ever want to find out.'

Jones Jr, a 1988 Olympic silver medallist, had yet to

encounter any kind of crisis in his career, let alone suffer a loss. He was often too quick to get hit, too fluid, too good, and to watch Jones Jr and Garcia in action was to almost watch two different sports, so different were their approaches, so alarming was the disparity in physical gifts. Gloves were the only commonality.

'Walk this guy down,' said Goossen to Ruelas before round seven. 'Get your hands up and push him. Walk through this punk. He don't want no part of you.'

HBO's Larry Merchant was more impressed. 'You can see some of the fire in this fighter,' he said while admiring replays of Ruelas' handiwork in between rounds. 'He wants to land punches with mean intentions. He wants to do damage. You're looking for that in a champion.'

Rounds seven and eight featured a different guy. This guy was bored, distracted, sulking. He was also now suddenly being outworked by the same modest challenger who was weight-drained, weak and unable to generate power in his punches.

'It says Jimmy Garcia has twenty-five knockouts, but it's hard for me to figure out how he got these knockouts,' wondered Jones Jr.

'They were all in his native Colombia,' said Lampley.

Knowing he couldn't be hurt, Ruelas frequently retreated to the ropes and let Garcia attack him. This new approach, born of frustration, allowed the challenger to throw a whopping 118 punches in round eight. No, not one of them made an impression, but they were point-scoring punches nonetheless and Ruelas, like a morose teenager, was now stuck in a funk from which he needed to escape. Yet he did just the same in round nine, only for longer; two minutes were spent on the ropes, from where he'd beckon Garcia in with a wave of his right glove, let him tickle him with jabs and body shots, and then look to spring off the ropes and unload explosive counter-punches. 'This is a frustrated fighter in Ruelas and I don't like what he's doing,' said Merchant. 'It doesn't make a lot of sense. He's bored and he's trying to amuse himself here.'

After spending most of the round against the ropes and in the corner, Ruelas *finally* moved.

'I felt I was winning decisively, but I told myself the fight wouldn't end unless I knocked him out,' he remembers. 'I thought, okay, I guess I'll just have to keep beating him up, and that was a horrible thing to think. I was worried because some of the shots I hit him with were sickening. I replay them in my mind even now. He just wouldn't go down. I wished he would go down every time I landed a punch on him.'

The final minute of round ten was the worst, as Ruelas allowed Garcia to touch him with jabs while on the move and then timed a slow jab and landed his own overhand right and left hook. He watched Jimmy sink into the ropes. 'He should stop this fight,' said Jones Jr, concerned, signalling to the referee, Mitch Halpern. 'This guy is very hurt. His legs are gone. Somebody should stop the fight. This guy is finished.'

Of the belief that Garcia's corner and Halpern would allow the massacre to continue, Ruelas did the only thing he knew. The one thing he was trained to do. He continued smashing heavy punches into a wounded opponent. Right hands over the top, body shots and uppercuts in the clinch, left hooks from out wide, they all landed, and a hook and right-cross combination on the bell appeared to shatter Garcia's jaw, for it swelled instantly. Larry Merchant, aghast, had seen enough of the slaughter. 'This is a fight that should be ended now,' he said as he watched Garcia struggle to navigate his way back to his corner. 'It doesn't look as if Garcia has any chance of turning it around. He's hurt, he's far, far behind and there really is no point in going on with this fight.'

As Manuel Jr held him by the ears and shook his head, perhaps to somehow regenerate him, ringside physician Dr Edwin 'Flip' Homansky of the Nevada State Athletic Commission joined referee Halpern in looking long and hard at Jimmy Garcia in his corner. They studied him as if analysing a painting for signs of forgery. But Jimmy, water running down his face, clocked their concern and said, 'I'm fine.'

'I remember thinking he shouldn't be in the ring with me any more,' says Ruelas. 'He was just a punch bag for me. I was hitting him over and over again and my hands had even started to hurt. That was something I'd never felt in any of my other fights. I'd never had hand problems in the gym or in the ring. But I hit Jimmy so often and so hard that my hands were in pain. They'd gone sort of numb. I never in a million years thought I'd one day be in the ring worried about hurting some guy. But I was. It happened that night.'

Believing a fighter's words, that he was fine, the corner of Jimmy Garcia let him go out for round eleven. But a left hook and two right hands later and Jimmy again sagged along the ropes, driven back by pure momentum and a loss of his own faculties rather than the ferocity of the punches, and Halpern waved it off with barely thirty seconds gone in the round.

'I don't like to see stuff like this,' said Jones Jr during the closing moments.

'I don't, either,' said Lampley.

Ruelas, the victor, barely raised his hands. The unhappiest winner of all time, he offered only a shrug and a half-smile as he toured the ring, head bowed, in what appeared to almost be a walk of shame.

'In some pictures, you could see me going to the other corner, the referee in the background is holding Jimmy, and I look like I lost the fight,' says Gabe. 'I look very sad. Maybe subconsciously I knew something bad had happened that night. I didn't know Jimmy was going to die. Nobody knew he was going to die. So I should have been happy at that moment, right? I should have been proud that I'd dominated the fight, defended my belt and finally got a stoppage. But in that picture, I look like the loser. That's really how I felt. It was one of my biggest wins but also my biggest loss.'

Master of ceremonies Michael Buffer took it upon himself to try and change the mood of the place. He snatched the microphone and bellowed, 'Ladies and gentlemen here at Caesars Palace, before I give the official time, how about a round of applause for the courage shown by this young challenger from Barranquilla, Colombia, Jimmy Garcia!' Applause rightfully followed and Goossen pointed for Ruelas to go and congratulate his challenger on a brave effort.

'Maybe I shouldn't have hit him with this shot or that shot, maybe I shouldn't have had such bad intentions before the fight and during the fight,' says Ruelas. 'We were taught to throw hurtful shots and combinations in the gym, to the head and body, and I used those in the fight. I used them to try and hurt Jimmy Garcia. My intention going into the fight was to hurt him and make him quit so that I could defend my title.'

Jimmy Garcia collapsed shortly after receiving his well-earned round of applause from the Caesars Palace crowd. He slid down to the canvas, a position he'd heroically avoided all night, and then started drifting in and out of consciousness.

'He's awake, he's awake,' reassured Homansky as an oxygen mask was applied to the mouth of the fighter. 'Let's see how he does for one minute. He's talking to us. He's fine.'

Garcia moved the mask away with his hands, either voluntarily or involuntarily, prompting his chief second and father, Manuel, to tell him to leave it on. 'They're concerned now, as they should be, but they should've been concerned a minute or two earlier,' said Merchant. 'They should not have sent him out for that round.'

Next, Garcia could be seen shaking out the fingers on his vitiligo-inflicted right hand. They moved all at once, in a kind of fluttering motion, and it was hard to know whether it was a controlled movement, one instructed by a medical professional, or a mere reflex and sign his body was in the process of shutting down. Tellingly, as a white stretcher was slid beneath the ropes and into the ring, Garcia, eyes closed, lost consciousness. 'He's fine, he's fine,' Homansky again reassured, but it was becoming harder to believe him. 'He's talking to us.'

'The fight went on too long,' cried a voice behind Homansky. 'Way too long. The last round that kid was hurtin' bad.'

Seven minutes after the fight was waved off, the frail, failing body of Jimmy Garcia was pushed into the back of a waiting ambulance. Before that he was carried through the flat Caesars Palace crowd, a scene resembling a funeral procession, and the fingers on his patchy brown-and-white hands continued to dance and reach out for something or someone beyond his grasp. Only now it was clear Jimmy's fingers weren't moving because he had been told to move them. They were moving because his brain was damaged.

THE DANGER
MAN I

This used to be his playground. It was where he came before fights, where he relaxed and where he 'knocked shit over'. But to reach his playground we must first shield our eyes from the searing neon lights of slot machines, an alligator-themed bar and a Mardis Gras-themed bar, and then dodge old age pensioners tired of the breakneck pace of the Strip who congregate around blackjack and poker tables, swigging from buckets of warm, syrupy Coca-Cola and marvelling at the giant heads of kings, queens and jesters, their eyes illuminated like the Zoltar Speaks fortune-teller machine in *Big*, which hang from the ceiling. It's Las Vegas. It's The Orleans Hotel & Casino. James Crayton, my forty-five-year-old tour guide in a white T-shirt two sizes too big for him, baggier red tartan shorts and scuffed-up sneakers, is familiar with the place. He boxed here thirteen times.

As I look around, however, I'm struggling to comprehend

fights, at least those of the organised variety, ever taking place in this worn-out establishment. Though it might be Vegas, the so-called 'fight capital of the world', it's hardly Caesars Palace. Far from it. This is the sort of place one winds up after crashing and burning on the Strip. This is purgatory, Vegas-style. Old men and women, as rusty as the machines into which they robotically pump coins and tokens, appear as though they've been here, awake, for days on end. The Mecca of Boxing? There's not a bicep in sight.

Crayton and I haven't come here to gamble. Nor have we come here to fight (though I inform him I'd like to see where he once boxed, if only to believe it actually exists). We have come here to visit the bowling alley he once frequented when, apprehensive and bored, he'd kill hours before a fight throwing balls down lanes and trying to connect with as many pins as possible. Nowadays, you see, Crayton – retired since May 2008 – is all bowler. He doesn't box any more. He has no interest in it, aside from watching others fight on television, and derives greater pleasure from playing on his bowling team every Friday night in El Rancho, Texas, ten miles from his home in Henderson. The team have no name, he tells me, but are a team nonetheless.

The Orleans bowling alley, meanwhile, is where old guys come to replenish when their brains have been sufficiently fried by the bright lights downstairs. It's far quieter, far less neon, and you can sit down at tables without fear of losing everything you own. 'This is my spot, buddy,' James says, as we take a seat near one of the lanes. 'Nobody could beat me here.'

We pause for a moment and watch an old guy in a tennis cap, tight-fitting shirt and khaki shorts, socks pulled up to his knees, stumble towards the line and dump, in the truest sense of the word, a purple bowling ball on the wooden floor, creating a loud thud, before turning away and cursing as it drifts way, way left and ends in the gutter. Crayton, sipping a caramel cappuccino, laughs to himself. He then looks around at others and tries to spot familiar faces, men he might once have played and defeated.

'Hey,' he says to a hotel employee wearing a blue polo shirt and a wrist brace.

'Hey,' the man replies. 'How you doing?'

'Doing good,' says Crayton. 'This is my old bowling buddy.'

'Not much of a bowler any more, unfortunately,' he says, pointing to his wrist.

'What happened?'

'I got tendonitis in my wrist.'

'Oh, man.'

'I've got to take a couple of weeks off.'

'Do you still bowl?'

'Yeah, I bowl on Tuesdays. I haven't been bowling the last couple of weeks, though. I'm probably going to come back next week and see how I feel.'

'He was a young kid when I was fighting here,' James tells me.

'Yeah, I was *really* young,' answers his friend, rubbing his gut.

The employee leaves and James explains that he used to bowl with the guy's dad, who unfortunately passed away, when he was here getting ready for fights in the nineties. 'I'd come here beforehand and throw a couple of balls,' he says. 'I'd be staying here at the hotel so it was easy. They'd say, "You shouldn't be bowling," but I didn't care. They were worried I might pull a muscle or something. But it relaxed me.'

The bowling bit I could believe. Crayton knew enough folk around these parts, on the lanes, for me to accept he once hung out here and made his name. But it was the boxing part I was struggling to comprehend. 'They haven't had a fight here in a while,' he concedes. 'When we used to fight, we'd fight upstairs. The fights would be in one of the banquet rooms. They've probably got desks and shit up there now. It's probably completely different.'

'How many people would watch?' I ask.

'I used to get at least fifteen hundred in there,' he says. 'When I fought main event, I sold it out. I had a big following, believe it or not. I was surprised when I'd fight in different countries and people knew who I was. I once went to Argentina to fight and fans there knew who I was. I even got fan mail from time to time. It was crazy.'

Maybe so, but 'Too Sweet' Crayton is still, despite the pen pals, one of the forgotten fighters of the nineties. His own spotlight dimmed, he was a durable, sometimes dangerous measuring stick used to gauge the potential of others, a high-end journeyman whose roll call of opponents includes former world champions Stevie Johnston, John John Molina, Julio Díaz, Javier Jáuregui, Derrick Gainer, Andre Berto and Gabriel Ruelas.

I tell him I've recently interviewed Ruelas and he knows what I'm going to say before I say it. 'Never the same after Jimmy Garcia, right?'

I nod my head. He shakes his.

'I don't like to talk about him, because it's not my place, but we fought something like eight months after he killed Jimmy and, I'm telling you, he was damaged. I could tell he was damaged when I was in the ring with him. He didn't fight like he used to fight.'

'How so?' I ask.

'He rocked me in something like the fourth round but never tried to follow up or do any more damage. He let me come back and I nearly knocked him out in the tenth round. I thought I won that fight. A lot of people thought I won that fight. Back then, though, my name wasn't as big as his name, so he got the benefit of the doubt.'

'Could he still punch hard?'

'Oh, he could still punch, don't get me wrong. They say the last thing you lose is your power and it's true. He still had that if nothing else. I was in there, thinking, okay, he's decent and he can punch, but this ain't the same guy I've been watching on TV for years.'

He stops there. I detect he wants to let Gabe tell his own story and doesn't feel comfortable doing so on his behalf. Changing lanes, he goes to great lengths to convince me his own professional boxing record of 34–28–2 is deceiving and that he not only deserved to beat Ruelas but also Díaz, Jáuregui and Ivan Robinson. Robbed, he claims, not once but four times. His was that kind of career. But, equally, Crayton is honest enough to accept he got a lucky draw against Stanley Longstreet, here at The Orleans, concedes that IBF world super-featherweight champion John John Molina was the best guy he ever faced, and goes on to say Pedro Saíz, the Dominican he battled in 1999, was the hardest-hitting. 'We fought here,' he recalls. 'He knocked me down in the first round with a flash knockdown. He caught me to the side of the head. Then, in the second round, I walked into something horrible. I was like, *goddamn*. I felt it go all through my body. Man, that shit was nasty. I still won the fight, though.'

Outside of competition, he says the person who punched him the hardest was Kostya Tszyu, the former undisputed world light-welterweight champion who Crayton sparred numerous times at the Top Rank gym in Vegas. 'Man, he could punch like a motherfucker,' he says. 'He lined me up for that right hand and when it landed I was seeing kookaburras, clocks and everything else. He could really crack.'

Born in Dallas, Texas, and raised between there and Vegas, Crayton wouldn't know a thing about his father until he was sixteen, as his mother left it to his grandmother and aunt to effectively bring him up, and he wouldn't know much about boxing until he was eighteen. But after hooking up with his coach, Pat Barry, a police officer, James won forty-eight of fifty-four bouts as an amateur and turned professional on 7 April 1994 with a two-round mauling of Agustín Rocha at the Silver Nugget here in Vegas. He'd go one better nine days later, crushing Mario Martínez in the first round at Caesars, and it wasn't long before he was getting busy. *Real busy*. Nine fights in 1994 and eleven in 1995. Any time, any place, he just wanted to get paid.

Still, before Crayton slipped into the role of trial horse for the stars, there were some noteworthy wins – yes, *wins* – on his professional record. Wins that should be celebrated, wins that hint at the danger he once possessed in his right hand. Take, for instance, his August 1995 victory over Saul Durán, 18–1 at the time and a future world title hope, who was flattened inside a round in Los Angeles. 'Oh, man,' says Crayton, rubbing his hands together, keen to get down to it. 'So, I went to LA to fight Durán and the inspector was fucking with me...'

'What do you mean?' I ask, worried I've misheard.

He gives me a look as if to say 'I'd explain if you let

me', so I let him. He takes us back to his dressing room at the Olympic Auditorium on the night of 24 August 1995.

'Why are you wearing coloured socks?' asked the inspector.

'My colours are red and black,' explained Crayton. 'It matches my uniform.'

— The inspector shook his head, perplexed. 'You should know the dye, when your foot sweats, will get in your foot and you can lose your foot,' he said.

'What?' said Crayton. 'Shut up, man.'

'Where's your mouth piece?'

'In my bag.'

'Take it out.'

Crayton did as he was told. He removed his mouth piece from his bag, slipped it into his mouth and took it out again, unsure of the reasons why. Shortly after that he was told to wrap his hands. Then he heard the words, 'Crayton, it's your turn.'

'Nah,' said Crayton. 'It ain't time for me to fight yet.'

He'd barely wrapped his hands and gloved up, let alone warmed up.

'I got into the ring and Pat, my trainer, was scared,' Crayton recalls. 'He said, "Are you okay?" I said, "They've been fucking with me, man. I want to knock this guy the fuck out. I want to kill this motherfucker."'

In round one Saul Durán was hit so hard by a right hand that had it not been for Crayton's body rudely interrupting the fall he'd have landed face-first on the canvas. True to his word, Crayton knocked him the fuck out.

This, by the way, is a phrase he likes: knocked the fuck out; K.T.F.O. It is, from his perspective, a term that best illustrates both his fighting *modus operandi* and the ultimate kind of victory. One that is definitive. One that lives in the memory. A knockdown from which there is no coming back.

Yet these animalistic urges threatened to desert Crayton following a fight with 'Jumpin'' Johnny Montantes on 26 September 1997, a fight that took place in a ring located somewhere inside The Orleans Hotel & Casino, a fight that, Crayton believes, should never have been arranged. 'Why the fuck have they let this guy fight me?' he asked himself time and time again during training camp and on fight day, too, when he sauntered around the hotel, threw some bowling balls to relax and eventually began warming up in a dressing room.

Crayton had never felt better going into a fight. Never stronger, never fitter, never faster, never more dangerous. It was partly for this reason he knew Johnny Montantes, a twenty-eight-year-old from Saint Paul, Minnesota, was in way over his head.

'When they announced Montantes was going to fight me, I was very surprised,' he says. 'This was a guy who previously turned down three contracts and told people, "I can't beat this man. He's too much on his game." Now, if a fighter tells you he can't beat someone, he's beaten already. The worst thing you can do is force him to take a fight he doesn't think he can win.'

Even more surprising for Crayton was the timing of it all. Montantes, understand, was hardly coming into the scheduled fight in a rich vein of form. On the contrary, he'd just suffered the third loss of his professional career, this time by first round knockout to Brazilian puncher Acelino 'Popó' Freitas, and was decked three times in the process. Worse still, it occurred only four months before he was slated to fight Crayton in Vegas.

'If you get knocked out badly like that you should be fighting someone who can't punch and who is easily moveable,' says James. 'There was no way in hell he was going to win. He was in too deep. It was almost impossible for him to beat me.'

Unlikely a view shared by Montantes at the time, he'd have pointed to the eight defeats on Crayton's record as eight reasons why he could feasibly prevail over ten rounds. Make no mistake, he was coming to win. He had even permanently moved to Las Vegas with his fiancée, Tammy Brunette, for the sole purpose of taking fights, winning fights and gradually progressing to a title shot.

Indeed, on the night of the fight, Montantes spread out the clothes he planned on wearing to the post-fight victory party on his hotel bed. They were ironed and prepared and he couldn't wait to wear them once the fight was over and the win was his. Those were the moments he did it for. Those small, priceless moments. Tammy and their two children, four-year-old Marciano and two-year-old Santino, would arrive later and bring with them flowers and a bottle of shoe polish. They too were invited to the party.

One man who wasn't was James Crayton. To him, the invitations were redundant. And that Friday night he fought with all the bitterness of someone turned away at the door.

'I couldn't miss,' says Crayton, a smile on his face. 'Nothing missed.'

Crayton's smile reveals a lot. It's a smile I associate with ego, particularly the ego of an athlete. He believes his handiwork, regardless of its consequences, is something to be admired. It brings him joy. Which is why, even when dealing in the macabre, the process of talking me through one of the most distressing nights of his life, Crayton can't help but describe the details, the mechanics, with a perverse sense of pride; accustomed to fighting superior men at late notice, this was, lest we forget, arguably the finest night of James Crayton's career; he was never better, never stronger, never fitter, never faster, never more dangerous.

'The first round I danced around the ring and, in my opinion, he shaded that one,' Crayton continues. 'In the second round, though, I just took over the fight. He was getting hit by right hands, left hooks, body shots... dude, it wasn't nice.'

Crayton shakes his head. Now he's serious, his voice less animated.

'In the sixth round (records indicate the bout ended in round five but Crayton, having double-checked, maintains it was round six) I threw an up-jab, cut him over the eye and Kenny Bayless, the referee, called "time". Now, I'd have been satisfied if they stopped the fight there and then. There was no way in hell he was going to win. He was getting beat up. But, as a fighter, you see red and go in for the kill.'

A shrug follows and his eyes appear to say, 'What the fuck was I supposed to do?' No longer does he seem proud. 'I go in, I nail him with a right hand and – *bam* – he's dazed. He grabs me. Kenny breaks it up. We separate and I hit him with an overhand right again. He hasn't thrown a punch for at least a good minute. His defence is non-existent...' Crayton drops his hands by his sides to mimic this helplessness. 'Do they stop the fight?' he asks, rhetorically. 'I can't stop punching, though. If I stop, I'm quitting. So I hit him with another right hand and it makes him even more wobbly. Now he's running around the ring.'

Crayton's smile returns at the gravest of moments. He tells me he remembers the finishing combination as if it were delivered only moments ago. 'I throw a one–two, miss, close the gap and then connect on his chin – right there,' he points to the very tip of his own, 'and he was out before he hit the canvas. Done deal. It was over.'

He knows now that it really was.

'They say he died two days later. In my honest opinion, though, he died that night. Here's a man who is unconscious, who has a seizure right there on the canvas and never wakes up again. I go to the locker room and change clothes and he's still lying there. He never walked out the ring. He never walked again.'

Though medical professionals told him otherwise, Crayton knew enough about his right hand, and the power it possessed, to discern this was no ordinary knockout. 'Oh, I knocked out a lot of people in my career – amateur, sparring, pro – and that one felt a *whole* lot different,' he says. 'When I hit him I literally felt it shoot up my arm. It was bone on bone. It made a horrible sound. They said, "Oh, don't worry, it's not your fault." Okay, you say it's not my fault, but had he not fought me, who knows, he could still be living today. We don't know that. I only know it was never my intention to kill a person.'

10

THE MASOCHIST II

Gabriel Ruelas knew he was a different Gabriel Ruelas the moment he got back from Las Vegas and informed his wife, Leslie, he was heading to the San Fernando Valley and that he'd return later. No time frame was put on this spontaneous voyage, nor did he feel any kind of elaboration or explanation was necessary. He fed his wife some bullshit about going to visit his mum and other family members, many of whom lived that way, but the truth was he had no idea what he was really planning on doing. He figured he'd drive around for a bit, see how far his wheels would take him, and then decide what to do when he got bored of pointlessly meandering.

Gabe sensed Leslie was worried, he could see it in her eyes, but he also believed this was something he needed. Ever since returning from his fight in Las Vegas, he yearned to get away again. There was a feeling of being suffocated at home. Too many news reports, too many pictures, too many questions. Yet nobody, he told himself, could get to him in the car. There'd be no contact, no phone calls, no curious glances directed his way. It would just be him, a steering wheel and the open road.

As it turned out, the new Gabriel Ruelas' first port of call was a car dealership. He justified the visit by reminding himself that his wife had just given birth to their first son, Diego, and that he desperately needed to get his hands on a more robust vehicle that could protect both of them. But no amount of rationalising could disguise the fact the old Gabriel Ruelas would never have done something so spontaneous, something so downright selfish. Normally, he says, if such a thought ever crossed his mind, he'd immediately call Leslie, discuss the idea with her, and then together they would assess their options and maybe – *maybe* – think about making a purchase. That was then. This was now. The new Gabriel Ruelas functioned differently to the old one. He didn't require Leslie's input to do the deal. He didn't even make the phone call. Rather, the young fighter, who came from nothing in the mountains of La Yerbabuena, paid the $70,000 asking price and took the keys to a brand-new truck. 'I just wanted to do something different,' he says now.

The new Gabriel Ruelas drove his new truck all the way home that evening and was accosted by Leslie, hands on hips, a frown stretched across the breadth of her forehead. 'What the hell are you doing?' she asked him.

'This is where I went,' he said. 'I went to buy a car.'

'Really? At this time of all times?'

Ruelas bowed his head. 'I know,' he said. 'I'm just trying to get away from it, I guess. I wanted to escape.'

The memories of his 6 May fight with Jimmy Garcia followed him all the way to the valley. He remembered the punches, the sounds, the damage, the collapse. He remembered ninety minutes after the fight going to the hospital with Leslie and being sat silent in the waiting room feeling a huge degree of guilt. He remembered not being allowed to see Jimmy until Jimmy's father had vouched for them. He remembered Jimmy's lips and head being swollen. He remembered everything because he saw and experienced everything. He really did. Ruelas fully immersed himself in the misery, as if wanting to punish himself, and bled alongside Jimmy. He too let it all out. The nurses and neurosurgeons at the University Medical Center knew him by name and he went out of his way to ensure the Garcia family were looked after and their medical and hotel bills were paid.

'Boxing is one of the hardest sports,' Manuel Jr, Jimmy's brother and trainer, told the *Los Angeles Times*. 'Sometimes you win, sometimes you lose. Sometimes you get a knockout and sometimes you get knocked out. You can lose your life in the ring. Fighters know this can happen. It was an accident. It was nobody's fault. We don't feel any bad towards him (Ruelas). He's a good sportsman. The way it happened to my brother, it could have happened to him, too.'

It took some time, however, for Carmen Garcia, Jimmy's mother, to come around to the idea that Gabriel Ruelas, her son's opponent, was now hanging around hospital wards and waiting rooms. At first, on the Monday, nine days after the fight, she declined to see him, turning her back on him completely, only for Gabe to respond by speaking to her in Spanish. A plea for forgiveness, at the very least it got her talking.

'I want to see you, but it has been hard for me because those hands hurt my son,' she said.

'I understand what you say,' he replied, 'because I feel guilty, but nobody can change what happened. As fighters, I believe all of us know the risks when we get into the sport.'

Carmen explained how she had warned her son about the threat of Gabriel Ruelas and had advised him not to fight the champion. 'In Colombia,' she said, 'they say you have knives in your hands.'

Gabe shook his head.

'They say you cut up fighters bad in the face.'

Gabe told her this was untrue. He said he never deliberately tried to inflict pain on an opponent in such a way.

'It didn't matter anyway,' she continued. 'He kept telling me, "Mom, I'm going to win the title, no matter what. I'm going to buy you a house. I was born to be a fighter. I would rather die than leave boxing."' Carmen then turned to look Gabe dead in the eye. 'Why didn't you let him win, Ruelas?' she asked. '*You* already won the title.'

An hour later, they were still talking, still crying, and then Carmen gave Gabe something far greater than words of comfort. She enveloped him with a hug. 'From now on,' she said, 'whenever you fight, I will see my son in you.'

It wasn't only Carmen's forgiveness Gabe sought during that difficult period. He'd also spend time by Jimmy's bedside, touching his hand, telling him how sorry he was. 'You know I didn't do this intentionally,' he said. 'I would give everything I have for you to stand up. I know you can't speak to me, but I wish you could give me a sign so that I will know you understand I didn't do it on purpose.'

Up to this point, Garcia had only moved the fingers on his left hand, but Ruelas' words somehow caused his left arm to suddenly jerk up and then drop back to his side. Gabe's initial reaction was one of delight, for it surely showed Jimmy had heard and forgiven him, but later he began to doubt that theory and instead wondered whether Jimmy was mad at him and that the left arm reacting the way it did was in actual fact an attempt to grab hold of him. Spooked, Gabe never told the doctors about the incident. Nor did he ever see Jimmy again.

Thirteen days after their fight, on 19 May 1995, doctors turned off the life-support system that had kept Jimmy Garcia's heart beating. There was nothing more they could do. His family were allowed a final chance to see him and then, shortly after, he was set free.

A part of Gabriel Ruelas went with Garcia that day and he has never been quite the same since. Once an extrovert full of life, inclined to have a good time and be around people, Gabe immediately went inside himself. He spent an increasing amount of time alone, thinking and mourning, and it became a strain to even smile. He felt guilty for doing so. There was guilt, too, attached to thoughts of a return to the ring.

'Most definitely I thought I'd never fight again,' he says. 'But after days, weeks and months, going through everyday life, you see the necessities your family needs and you realise you're stuck with this. I had no choice. I had to fight because it was my job. You can't just quit your job when something bad happens. It was what I chose to be. It was what I had dedicated my whole life to. I had to continue.'

Seven months after the Garcia tragedy, Ruelas was asked to defend his WBC world super-featherweight title in a rematch with Azumah Nelson, the pay-per-view proceeds of which would be donated to a trust fund Gabe was setting up for the three young children Garcia left behind. It was a tough fight on paper for the old Gabriel Ruelas, having lost a majority decision to Nelson in February 1993, but the new Gabriel Ruelas was no match for the Ghanaian in December 1995. This time it wasn't even competitive. Nelson stopped Gabe in five rounds. He was no longer a world champion. 'I knew I was a different person,' he says. 'I used to go in there and want to beat guys up so bad. I'd want to hurt them. To motivate myself, I'd look at videos of Mike Tyson and watch his quick knockouts over and over. I'd think of him before fights and want to hurt guys the way he hurt them. But that completely stopped after Jimmy Garcia. It didn't work for me any more. I was careful of landing punches. That's something you can't do in this business because you can end up getting hurt yourself.'

Getting hurt never bothered Ruelas. In 1997, Arturo 'Thunder' Gatti knocked him out in seven rounds in a classic. A year later, John Brown halted him in eight. Courtney Burton then did the same in 2003, after which Ruelas called it a day. Bizarrely, each time he was hit and hurt, each time he was knocked down or knocked out, Gabe told himself it was God's way of punishing him for what he had done to Jimmy Garcia at Caesars Palace. 'That's why I wanted to fight,' he says. 'I felt responsible, I felt it was my fault and I felt I should be punished for what I did. I could only find some sort of peace by getting hurt. I know that sounds crazy, but I wanted to get hurt in the ring just as Jimmy had been hurt. I needed to be punished for what I had done. I would fool everybody in training and look good and all that, but, when the fight came, it was time for what I wanted – I wanted to get hurt.'

Assuming he'd be dead at twenty-five, once Ruelas, now a

'train without brakes', passed that milestone, his life spiralled out of control. He became an alcoholic. He crashed his car multiple times. He did all he could to forget the past and shorten his future. The grim reaper stayed close, too, when Mitch Halpern, the third man in the ring the night Gabe defeated Jimmy Garcia, died on 20 August 2000 in his south Las Vegas home from a self-inflicted gunshot wound to the head. He was just thirty-three years old. Nobody knew why he did it, and few linked it back to the Jimmy Garcia tragedy, but, like Richard Green, Halpern was a Vegas-based referee involved in a Caesars Palace ring tragedy who one day decided to take his own life with a shotgun. Coincidence? All Gabe knows is that he could so easily have gone the same way. His drink of choice was tequila and most nights he'd neck two or three bottles and then flop down in a stupor, caring not whether he woke the next morning. 'When I don't drink, I don't know who I am,' says the man who has now swapped tequila for wine, claims to only drink at weekends, and has stopped driving altogether. 'When I'm drinking, I feel some kind of relief. It's therapeutic. I'm a very calm person. I'm relaxed. It's how I used to be. I'm always trying to find my old self.'

Eighteen years after Jimmy Garcia passed away in a Las Vegas hospital, Ruelas took the pilgrimage to his opponent's home city, Barranquilla, Colombia, with the intention of spending a few days with the Garcia family. The trip allowed him to meet Jimmy's two teenage daughters and son for the first time and for him to apologise to them just as he had once apologised to the other members of the family in Sin City. There was plenty of crying and heartfelt embraces when the Garcias reiterated to Gabe that they had never placed any blame at his door. They even submitted to him that Jimmy's medical history, kept quiet from the commission before the fight, flagged up issues he'd had with a previous bleed on the brain and that that, rather than Gabe's punches, could have been the main cause of the tragedy. They said doctors had informed Jimmy and his father of the problem, but both had chosen to ignore it. It left the rest of the family incensed when they found out. It offered Gabe, meanwhile, some form of relief. 'Closure,' he called it.

While in Barranquilla he got the chance to see Carmen again and this time there was no hostility. They hugged immediately. They sobbed into each other's arms. Gabe even took to calling her 'Nana', the title Jimmy Garcia had once bestowed upon her. She liked that. She wanted him to call her by that name. 'I have two mothers now,' said Gabe. 'If I could afford it, I would take you to Mexico so you could visit my other mom.'

As is his tendency, Gabe then suddenly lost his train of thought. He pictured his own mother and wondered how she would have felt if it had been Jimmy Garcia spending time with her in Mexico having killed her son. It was then that his words trailed off and his mind went blank. He shook his head clear. He smiled a hollow smile.

'I'm not fully okay with my role in what happened,' he says now. 'I don't blame myself as much after going to Barranquilla, but it was still me fighting him and punching him and hurting him. I was the one in the ring with him trying to knock him out. I also blame the commission, the doctors, the whole team. It's not just me. A lot of people were at fault for what happened to Jimmy Garcia. But I have to live with my role in it until the day I die, just as his kids have to live with the fact they won't have a father. I'll never feel completely innocent.'

11

THE THIRD MAN

He's supposed to be relaxing and taking his mind off boxing, but as he lounges in his Las Vegas home, days from fight night, referee Kenny Bayless imagines the two tennis players on his television screen as championship prizefighters. One leads off, the other counter-punches. One takes control, the other rallies back. They both dig in at various points, keen to gain the upper hand, and both will stop at nothing to advance to the next stage of the US Open.

Forever the referee, Bayless, perhaps the most famous third man in boxing today, alternates between watching the two tennis players. He analyses them, admires them. Beyond that, he studies the flow of the game, how it's handled by the umpire, how both players go about conquering the other. 'Sharpening my eyes,' he calls it. It doesn't matter whether it's boxing, tennis, basketball or football, Bayless uses sports, especially televised sports, to sharpen his eyes. If he misses something at home, there's no harm done. There's nobody to answer to. Get it wrong on fight night, however, and, well, that's a different story. 'Boxing isn't tennis, that's for sure,' he says with a chuckle, wanting to make the distinction totally clear. 'Oh, boy, you realise that pretty quickly. It's no game at all, in fact. No game at all.'

Born and raised in Berkeley, California, Bayless' obsession with boxing began when he watched Muhammad Ali fight on *Wide World of Sports*, then cranked up a notch when he moved to Las Vegas in 1972, having been recruited as a physical education school teacher, and started attending live boxing shows along the Strip. One day, in 1973, Ali came to town to fight Joe Bugner at the Convention Center and Bayless made sure he was there to witness his first live Ali appearance. It was, he reckons, love at first sight.

Kenny was the only Bayless to show an interest in boxing, though admits he comes from an athletically gifted family. When in college, he played some basketball, tennis and ran track, becoming an All-American in track and field, and even tried out for the 1976 Olympic team alongside his twin brother, Kermit. Kenny specialised in the 400 metres, while the two Bayless boys both tried out for the 4 X 400-metre relay team. The 1976 Olympic dream would ultimately prove a step too far, but boxing had a wider wingspan, thus more opportunity, and Kenny was embraced wholeheartedly when deciding to pursue judging roles in a Golden Gloves amateur tournament in 1977. He had by now cut his teeth as a judge, taking a pen and notepad to various shows in Las Vegas, unofficially scoring as many bouts as he could, and was also assisting a friend he knew at the Nevada State Athletic Commission who was responsible for sorting the boxers' gloves on fight night. 'That was my way in,' says Bayless, who was then later asked to consider refereeing. At first his instinct was to turn down the opportunity. He didn't believe he knew enough about the sport to be deemed responsible for the well-being of two fighters. But he gave it some thought, allowed the idea to marinate, and then confronted legendary referee Richard Steele, who assured him he had the goods. Together, Richard and Kenny went to different gyms, watched sparring sessions, interrupted sparring sessions, and discussed hypothetical situations, working through the many dos and don'ts along the way. In 1982, Kenny began refereeing amateur bouts when he wasn't judging them. 'It was definitely a learning experience because you really have to train your eye,' he says.

Bayless officially refereed his first pro bout, a four-rounder between Ka-Dy King and Derrick Edwards, on 9 April 1992 at Bally's, Las Vegas. He refereed his first world title fight in 1994, a WBC world minimumweight title fight between Ricardo López and Surachai Saengmorakot, and has gone on to be the third man in over a hundred world title contests around the globe. It wasn't until 2004, though, that he believes he finally made it as a high-profile referee. That was the year he was given his first super-fight, the world middleweight title encounter between Bernard Hopkins and Oscar De La Hoya, and courted derision from sports analysts who didn't feel he was experienced enough to handle such an occasion. Marc Ratner, the executive director of the Nevada State Athletic Commission, thought otherwise. He said Bayless, someone who overcame a prostate cancer diagnosis in 2003, was categorically the right man for the job. His decision was final.

'When two fighters get in the ring, it's all about our ability to stay focused,' says Bayless, who, at sixty-five, hikes, bikes, and runs when he can, often using a treadmill in his Vegas home. 'We have to have three minutes of total concentration regardless of what happens. We have to be prepared for what may come. People ask me, "Do you watch tape on fighters?" Well, yes we do. We watch tape and we teach. In a lot of our seminars we go over certain situations that might crop up. We work out what to do and how to respond to them. You're never too old to learn.'

It's this attention to detail which sees Bayless, a father of three [James, Kenny Jr and Alex], keep getting the big assignments. It's why, in May 2015, he was asked to referee the so-called biggest fight in history between Floyd Mayweather Jr and Manny Pacquiao; the Nevada State Athletic Commission considered five other referees for the fight but appointed Bayless by a unanimous 5–0 vote. 'I can't believe it,' Leonard Ellerbe, CEO of Mayweather Promotions, said to the *Los Angeles Times*, 'but this is one thing [Pacquiao promoter] Bob Arum and I *do* agree on. We're very pleased with the selection of the officials. The referee will undoubtedly do a masterful job.'

So highly regarded was Bayless, in fact, and so grand was the event, he earned a record $25,000 for the assignment, more than any other boxing referee in history (put in context, Mayweather stood to make the same sum, $25,000, in around three-tenths of a second of a fight expected to generate as much as $500 million in total revenue).

Now, as he prepares to officiate yet another Mayweather fight – this time a September 2015 vanity project against Andre Berto, for which Bayless will be paid a comparatively paltry $10,000 – he often spares a thought for Johnny Montantes, just as he spares a thought for Pedro Alcázar and Martín Sánchez, two other men he watched transition from athletic specimens to comatose victims before his very eyes. For Bayless, there have been many world title fights, a handful of so-called super-fights and, yes, three ring tragedies. He oversaw Fernando Montiel's sixth-round stoppage of Alcázar at the MGM Grand in 2002, and then three years later watched as Rustam Nugaev beat up Martin Sánchez at The Orleans Hotel & Casino. Both ended in tragedy. His first, though, was the 1997 battle between James 'Too Sweet' Crayton and 'Jumpin'' Johnny Montantes. 'It was a real strange fight,' he remembers. 'The fighter who hit the fighter that ultimately died was not known to have a knockout punch. He was the kind of fighter that would take you the distance as opposed to having this big knockout punch.'

Confused, I ask Bayless whether the James Crayton in question is the same James Crayton I'd spent a few hours getting to know in Vegas. Turns out it was. If so, it seems remiss of Bayless to describe him as a light-hitting fighter, especially when a significant number of his wins back then were decided by knockout; thirteen knockouts from twenty-three wins going into the Montantes fight is a reasonable return by anyone's standard.

'When Crayton hit his opponent,' Bayless continues, 'you could see the lights turn out. When he hit the ground, I didn't even think to start counting. His head hit the canvas and his body totally shut down.'

'Did you know it was serious at that point?' I ask.

'Yes,' he says. 'I knew he was going to be in a serious condition because when he went down and I waved the fight off I looked into his eyes and could see how glassy they were. They were kind of rolling back a little bit. At that point you just pray and hope he survives. In that case, he didn't.'

DOG ROUNDS

Johnny Montantes' left pupil was pinpointed, meaning there was a haematoma on the right side of the brain, and he went into a seizure. Ringside physicians Robert Voy and Charles Signoreno, as well as Nevada State Athletic Commission chairman Dr Elias Ghanem, treated him in the ring, administering oxygen and intravenous fluids, but he lapsed into a coma before being taken out of the ring on a stretcher. Nineteen minutes later, a waiting ambulance crew had him in the emergency room at University Medical Center, the same hospital in which Jimmy Garcia was treated.

Neurosurgeon John Anson operated at UMC and blood was drained from the area between Montantes' brain and skull, yet he remained in critical condition until declared clinically brain dead on the Sunday at around 1:30p.m., less than forty-eight hours after his fight with Crayton. His family agreed to donate his organs and his fiancée, Tammy, tried to establish a memorial fund for their sons, Marciano and Sonny, aware that Johnny had no life insurance and that his $2,000 fight purse combined with the $50,000 death insurance (under Nevada regulations boxers have a $50,000 accidental death benefit) wouldn't last long.

'When he passed, they told his fiancée she would get fifty grand for the funeral and their kids' college fees or whatever,' says Crayton, who attended a small funeral arrangement for Montantes at a Vegas church before his body was taken back to Minnesota. 'You know as well as I do fifty thousand dollars ain't going to replace a life. Fifty grand ain't shit. The sad thing is he lost his life for two thousand dollars. He fought me for two grand. That's fucking peanuts.

'As a fighter, though, you know what you're getting into. Before you even sign that contract, it tells you right there that there's a chance that death could happen or you could

148

get severely hurt. It's down to us, as fighters, to choose whether we want to do it or not. Nobody forces us. I signed my waiver. I was prepared for it. So was he.'

Bayless received the news at roughly the same time as everyone else – that Sunday afternoon – and reacted the way they all did. He shed tears, he asked questions of himself and he wondered whether or not he wanted to continue being involved in such an unforgiving business. 'It was tragic,' he says. 'That's all there is to it. When I got the call, I was inconsolable. I cried over and over. I asked myself, "Is this a sport I want to be a part of? Do I want to be known as a boxing referee?" People die in this sport.'

Having spoken to Crayton while in Vegas, I knew he placed some of the blame on Bayless, if not all of it. He accepted the fact the ending was as swift as it was definitive, and that little was known about either man going in, but still he would have liked to have seen the referee jump to the stoppage before it was too late. I could tell that irked Crayton even now, all these years later.

'He [Montantes] was taking a hell of a beating from the second round on,' recalls Crayton, 'but in the sixth round it went bad. Once he got that cut, it was all downhill. You see guys getting beaten up badly and they're too brave to quit. This was like that. You just think, someone step in and save the guy. Just stop it. We got to that point and I don't know why nobody helped him.'

Understandably, Bayless is more philosophical about it.

'The number-one thing, when we're in our seminars and talking as a group, is the safety of the fighter,' he says. 'We watch a lot of film and decide at what point you should become concerned about the amount of punishment a fighter's taking. There are also certain things we'll do between rounds. We'll go over and say a few words to the fighter. We'll get the fight doctor in the ring and let them analyse him. If we see a guy has taken too much, the trigger goes off and you don't second-guess it. You stop it. That trigger is hard-wired into your subconscious. It's the result of officiating and watching many, many fights. You don't even think about the decision. You just know. I have never gone back and thought I should have stopped a fight sooner than I did. With Montantes, there wasn't anything I could do because it was a one-punch knockout. I didn't even have a say in the matter. It was just a one-punch thing.'

The trigger never went off the night Crayton ended the life of Montantes. That's not to say it should have gone off, nor is it to say Bayless did a bad job – too much grey area makes either assertion unfair – but what we do know is that Bayless, the man in charge, walked away from The Orleans Hotel & Casino on the night of 26 September 1997 satisfied with his own performance. He placed faith in his instincts and that night they were, in his view, as good as on any other night.

Which, I guess, begs the question, who, then, *is* to blame? Bayless, like the rest, has a theory.

'As referees,' he says, 'we don't know the history of the fighters. We don't know how easy or hard they found it making weight. We don't know what their training camp was like. We don't know if they got beat up in sparring. We don't even know if they have an underlying medical issue.

'They all come with passports and that passport helps the commission decide the rest they should have between fights. In the case of Montantes, he was coming off a first-round knockout defeat in his previous fight and returned four months after this knockout. You don't know if something in that fight could have caused something to happen against Crayton. It could have gone undetected for all we know. Whether that had any bearing on matters, I don't know. Those are the kind of things that are beyond our control. We're not matchmakers. We haven't put these two men together.'

Although their views may differ, Bayless and Crayton were arguably the two men – beyond the victim's family – most affected by what happened to Montantes. They were certainly the closest to it. The closest two to death. Kenny, in particular, has been closer than us all to some of the grisliest knockouts in the history of the sport and is subsequently without the benefit of the soft focus lens through which the rest of us watch an art we deem noble.

'The Montantes death was tough on everyone involved,' he says. 'Personally speaking, I didn't know if I wanted to continue refereeing any more. Luckily, I had a good team of referees around me, including Richard Steele, and they supported me. Marc Ratner was the executive director at the time and he said, "I'm going to put you in on our very next fight. This is something you have to get over. It happens in our sport. You can do everything by the letter and these things still happen." I was able to go back in the ring shortly after and put that behind me.'

Bayless feels the biggest mistake he has made so far as a referee is when he got out of position and a little complacent and called a push by Shane Mosley on Manny Pacquiao a knockdown. A count was administered, Pacquiao appeared perplexed and the Las Vegas crowd were up in arms. But Bayless knows why now. He saw the replays, he canvassed opinion. He knew he had screwed up. 'I'm just as human as anyone else and I've done it,' he says. He felt bad enough afterwards to apologise to Pacquiao for getting the call wrong. 'It happens.'

Pacquiao, as affable as any fighter in the modern era, simply smiled, shrugged and thanked Bayless for being so honest. It mattered not to him. He won the 2011 fight regardless. But referees who find themselves involved in ring tragedies aren't afforded the same opportunity when the fight ends and the dust settles. They don't get the chance to put it right.

'You never forget them,' Bayless says, 'and it doesn't require that type of situation for you to realise that every time you step in there you can never be sure what the outcome is going to be. All you can do is make sure you always bring your A-game. You just never know when you're going to get unlucky with one.'

12

THE DANGER MAN II

'I don't know if it's open or not,' he says as we approach a large door and his hand reaches for the long, metallic push bar. 'But, trust me, motherfuckers used to fight in here.'

Nearby signs tell us we've finally made it to the Mardis Gras ballroom, the room in which all fights at The Orleans Hotel & Casino have taken place over the years, and neither of us could be happier. I'm delighted to know it exists, having been sceptical all afternoon, and James 'Too Sweet' Crayton, once the darling of this establishment, is positively charged with fond memories, flashbacks and a sense of pride. He's one such motherfucker. Not only that, of the twenty-eight defeats on his professional boxing record, only one of them occurred here – decided on a cut, no less – so, in terms of happy hunting grounds, this is about as good as it gets. 'This was my home,' he confirms as the door opens and we stumble upon the room in which a man's life once ended.

DOG ROUNDS

Seemingly set up for some kind of conference, there are round white tables scattered all over the place, each of them accompanied by countless metal chairs, as well as trollies containing bins, and the ceiling is illuminated by a number of panel lights and chandeliers decorated with what appear to be autumnal leaves. Chandeliers aside, though, it's primarily a beige room, one fit only for men and women in suits being offered sparkling water and finger sandwiches from a tray, and it's a reminder, once again, that we're a long way from Caesars Palace. In fact, were it not for the former professional fighter stood in the middle of the room, with one finger raised as he poses for a photograph, you'd be hard pressed to find any indication that boxing matches ever took place here.

'The ring would be right there in the middle and there'd be seats all around it,' Crayton assures me. 'It would be standing room only. They'd have the projector screens on the wall right there so you could catch replays if everyone was stood up and you couldn't see the action.'

'Where would you walk to the ring?' I ask.

'From back there,' he says, pointing to the far end of the room. 'That's where the dressing rooms would be. It was a very short ring-walk. You'd stand right there until the music came on and then you'd make the walk. The atmosphere was crazy. I used to have this place on its toes, man.'

That I can believe. A room so small is surely ideal for temporarily homing hundreds upon hundreds of intoxicated gamblers keen to see two men beat the shit out of each other before they head back downstairs and lose more money at the tables.

'I reckon it might have been in the early 2000s when they last held an event here,' says Crayton. 'My last fight here was the Montantes fight, I think.'

He's wrong. I decide to tell him. 'No, you fought here many times after that.'

'Nah-ah. I didn't.'

'You did.'

'Really? Who'd I fight? I never lost here.'

He pauses for thought.

'Oh, shit, you're right,' he says. 'I fought [Ernesto] Zepeda here. That was a seventh-round stoppage.'

'See,' I say, happy to gloat. 'It really was a good-luck charm for you.'

'Ain't that the truth,' he says. 'Don't fight James Crayton here. Don't fight him, period. But *definitely* don't fight him here.'

Crayton's final fight in this room took place on 3 May 2002 and was indeed a seventh-round stoppage of Ernesto Zepeda. Something of a landmark, James would record only one more win between that date and the date of his retirement in 2008.

Sadly, after the Montantes tragedy, James Crayton became the very thing he always feared becoming. He became Gabriel Ruelas. Specifically, he became the faded, gun-shy version of the former WBC world super-featherweight champion he had faced in 1997.

His next loss, a July 1998 defeat to Golden Johnson, only served to emphasise the point.

'I was scared,' James says. 'I can count on one hand how many right hands I threw in that whole twelve-round fight. I threw five.'

By the fifth round, Eddie Mustafa Muhammad, the former WBA world light-heavyweight champion, said to Crayton in the corner, 'What's wrong with your right hand?'

'Nothing,' James said.

'Then how come you ain't throwing it?'

The fighter knew why he was unwilling to let it go, but how could he possibly explain it to anyone else? 'I was scared that if I hit this guy the same way I hit Montantes, then maybe the same shit would happen to me again. It would be like déjà-fucking-vu.'

Crayton won only seven of his next twenty-eight fights. Many he lost because he simply refused to throw his right hand. He knew it. The opponent knew it. Everyone did. Even his eight-year-old son, James Jr, could see what was happening to his hero.

'Dad, you don't fight the same no more,' James Jr said to his father one day.

'What do you mean?'

'You don't throw your right hand no more.'

'Huh?'

'Since you killed that guy, you don't really throw it.'

Crayton frowned, told his son he was worrying unnecessarily, but knew, deep down, he was right. 'Nah,' he said, 'Daddy's all right.'

But, really, he wasn't. There's nothing all right about losing the final eight fights of his career.

'People say, "But you've got twenty-four losses on your record." I say, "Yeah, but it doesn't mean I was a bad fighter." Those twenty-four losses came from me letting people beat me. If you're going to be technical about it, I beat myself. If the right James Crayton showed up, I'd have kicked ass. But I was done. I thought, this ain't for me any more. Why get hurt? It's a hard thing to accept but it's made easy when you're losing to people you know you would've destroyed at your best.'

Since retiring he has become a working man who watches

fights on television and goes bowling every Friday; his most recent job sees him make food trays for the elderly residents of the Canyon Vista Medical Center. Yet fond memories of the destruction caused by his right hand remain.

'God gave me that right hand,' he says. 'It's natural. It's my greatest possession. I never knew how good my right hand was until I was deep in my career. Before, when I was with Pat Barry, he taught me the basics, the one–twos and all that. When I got with Eddie Mustafa, though, it was like, okay, you can move, but now it's time to show you how to pivot and transfer your weight and stuff. He showed me how to put my punches together and how to hurt a person. Ironically, the Johnny Montantes fight was the first time me and Eddie Mustafa hooked up. It changed *his* life, too.'

For a moment, he wanders and I panic I've lost him. He ambles ahead, weaving in and out of tables, checking the floor space as though measuring for fresh carpet. Intrigued, I begin to follow. 'What is it?' I ask.

'Okay,' he says, stopping, hands on hips. He then points to the floor. 'If this is where the ring was – right here – then he probably landed right there.'

It's 'Jumpin'' Johnny Montantes, I tell myself, careful not to be heard. All that's missing is a chalk outline.

'I came around the corner,' Crayton says, mimicking the action with his raised right hand, 'I hit him – *boom!* – and he landed back like this and was literally lying right there in that spot. His head hit the canvas where your foot is.'

Feeling nauseous at the thought, I instinctively remove my foot from the spot and take a step back. I then watch Crayton shake his head. 'He was never conscious again,' he says. 'He took his last breath right there. September the twenty-sixth, 1997. I'll never forget it.'

Stunned by this ability to reconstruct one of the most harrowing moments of his fighting life in such graphic detail, I search for signs he is human. I ask him how he feels. I say how hard it must be for him to return here after so many years. I beg him to show me something. No, not more punches, James. *Something else.*

'Listen, man, when I started boxing, I said I wanted to make history. But not *that* way. This is nothing to brag about. It's not something I like talking about. I'm not proud of the fact I killed someone in the ring. But it's in the history books and that man will be connected to me for the rest of my life.'

That's better, I think. I can run with that. It makes the previous action, the re-enactment, less morbid.

'The people who work here won't even know that happened,' says Crayton, back to pacing. 'They've probably got new employees here now.'

By chance he catches the eye of one, an older black gentleman with grey hair and a bushy moustache, strolling with a trolley out in front of him.

'Excuse me, sir,' says James. 'How long have you been working here?'

'Two years,' replies the man.

'Oh, just two. You wouldn't know when they last did boxing here.'

The man nods with certainty. 'Two months ago,' he says. 'They had UFC [he means mixed martial arts] and then they had wrestling –'

'No, no, *boxing*,' says James, shaking his head.

'Oh, they had boxing this year. It was amateurs. They've always got something going on here. They've got UFC, they've got wrestling, some boxing. Why, you guys going to set something up in here?'

'No, I fought here many years ago. This is my home venue.'

'They had a boxing event in February, I think. It was only amateur, nobody big.'

'I used to fight here all the time. I was a household name here.'

The man's eyes light up. 'Oh, yeah?' he says. 'What's your name?'

'James Crayton.'

'James Crayton? Nice to meet you. I'm Danny Wallace.'

They shake hands.

'You guys just touring?'

'Yeah.'

'You done?'

'Yeah, I'm retired now.'

'You still seem like you've got your wits about you,' says Danny, tapping the side of his head with his index finger.

James laughs. He looks over at me. 'We were just talking about that.'

'They always said you guys suffer from concussions and slurred speech and all that.'

James laughs again, louder this time.

'You know what that means,' says Danny. 'You know how to bob-and-weave. You can get out the way. And you train properly.'

'It's funny, people say, "You don't look beat up, you don't talk funny, you don't walk funny." Yeah, it means I was a good fighter. If I don't have any bumps and bruises and I ain't all fucked up and shit, it means I was good at what I did.'

'Yeah, you weren't only offensive, you were *defensive*, too.' Danny puts up his hands and frantically shifts his head left and right. 'You knew how to protect yourself.'

'Exactly!' cries James. 'I really didn't get hit that much. I still have my faculties. I'm not punch drunk. My memory's great. I can still pass a neurological exam if I wanted to fight again.'

'Good to see you, man,' Danny says as they shake hands a second time.

'You too, man,' replies James. 'Good to know I ain't fucked up.'

Danny returns to his trolley and we head our separate ways. Outside the room there's a convention for hypnotists being set up. We predict they'll move into the ballroom later that day and Crayton, fascinated, can't help but ask a blonde woman on the front desk, presumably part of the admin staff, if she is able to hypnotise him there and then. Unsurprisingly, she can't. So we move along. 'Those tables would've been covered in posters and programmes back in the day,' James says with a sigh. 'It would've been "will call", you know, where you get your tickets.' Crayton kisses his teeth. 'Now look at it. Fucking hypnotists.'

We make our way back through the casino, rubbing bare shoulders with decrepit old men in vests and flip-flops, and end up roughly where we started. Then one of the automatic doors to the car park slides open and a surge of forty-five-degree desert heat engulfs my face and won't budge; even Crayton, a local, shakes his head in disbelief as he wipes the perspiration from his brow.

'Here,' he says, while I prepare a sweaty handshake, 'take a look at this.'

He floats his phone beneath my nose and hits play on a video clip of a black man knocking out a lighter-skinned man in a boxing ring.

'Who is that?' I ask.

'That's me knocking the fuck out of Saul Durán.'

He does exactly that. Just as he'd earlier explained to me.

'Not bad, huh?' he says, laughing. 'That was one of the best right hands I threw in my life.'

'There was no coming back from that,' I say, simply eager to contribute.

He fiddles with his phone some more, returns it to his chest, and then, once satisfied, holds it in front of me for a second time. Same thing again. I'm able to make out a black guy hunting down a white guy, landing heavy shot after heavy shot on his poor, unprotected head, but have nothing more to go on than that.

'Who's this?' I say.

'Montantes,' he answers.

'*Johnny* Montantes?'

'Uh-huh.'

A few seconds later I watch Crayton connect with the right hand that ended the life of 'Jumpin'' Johnny Montantes here at The Orleans Hotel & Casino eighteen years ago. The very same right hand that moments earlier, in the very same Mardi Gras ballroom, he re-enacted on the very same spot on the floor. It may as well be a clip of a beheading in the Middle East.

In a state of shock, I again analyse his face for clues. Clues as to how he feels. Clues he is human. Clues he cares. But, before I can collect the evidence and make any kind of assessment, he hits rewind on the clip and we watch the killer blow land a second time. This time my gulp is surely audible.

Perhaps the heat is to blame and that's why I watch. It has made me illogical, woozy and weak. Or maybe I convince myself it's important to know what *really* happened, to see it with my own eyes, rather than take someone's word as gospel. Right, James? And, let's be honest: each and every one of us would struggle to avert our gaze if put in the same position. Right? It's a knockout, after all. We *love* knockouts. Sure, it's unnerving to think Crayton carries this footage on his phone and is capable of showing it to anyone he seeks to impress, but, in fairness, he'd said already that he considered the punch and the performance to have been the best of his career, so why *wouldn't* he be proud of the achievement? To us, those made of softer stuff, it's a reminder of a great tragedy, yet, to him, the boxer, it's pure sport, it's the fight business, a demonstration of something he has done since childhood. Yeah, a guy died, but it wasn't necessarily his fault. Nor was it his intention. James Crayton only wanted to knock someone the fuck out. And, I guess, in his mind, that's exactly what happened.

His reaction should have come as no surprise. Earlier, when kicking back on the bowling lanes, Crayton revealed to me he has a DVD of the fight at home that he watches from time to time, though hasn't of late. It wasn't, he said, revisited for him to gloat or revel in another man's untimely downfall, but was instead watched because he wanted to spot the mistakes he and Montantes made and simultaneously admire the best performance and knockout of his up-and-down career. He explained, 'Even one of the judges told my trainer, "That's the best I've ever seen Crayton look."'

'What mistakes did Johnny Montantes make?' I had asked him.

'His biggest mistake was taking the fight,' replied Crayton. 'I wish they had protected him a bit more. But, in terms of the fight, he wasn't throwing the jab enough and he was throwing looping, wild shots I could see a mile away. I'm a smart fighter. I'm not a dumb fighter. I was able to just take away his best weapon, the left hook, and then go to work. He'd hit me with it once but then he wouldn't land it again.'

Back outside, phone returned to his pocket, I ask him, 'What will you do when you get home?'

'I'm gonna go play some PlayStation,' he says.

'Oh, that's good.'

'Yeah. I'm playing a lot of *Madden* [NFL] these days.'

'You like video games?'

'Uh-huh. Play 'em all the time.'

Forgoing sweaty handshake in favour of sweatier hug, he lets me know he'll send me a DVD of the Montantes fight to help add detail to what he has already told me and then he almost evaporates in the Vegas heat. It's unlikely I'll ever see him again, long-distance relationship and all that, so I thank him for the gesture – you know, helping with my research – and then thank him twice for being so honest. Almost *too* honest, I say.

I return to England and weeks and months pass and there's no DVD. I nudge him from time to time and ask, via phone call or text message, how far along he is in the process, but still nothing. One day he tells me he's uploading the necessary files to a disc, the next he tells me he's on his way to the post office to drop the thing off. There's always a logical reason for the delay. It all sounds good to me. It's why I continue to wait with bated breath, why I wonder each morning if today will be the day. If he's the drug dealer, I'm the fiend waiting for the next hit; that death match.

As time drags on, though, I come to terms with what it actually is I'm expecting from this man and question my need to see it all over again, this time on a bigger screen, all the while recalling how uncomfortable, sleazy and despicable I felt when Crayton flashed the finishing punch up on his phone in Sin City. In this instance, I conclude, the buyer is no better than the seller.

Still nothing. There's no sign of the DVD and I continue to rely on words rather than video evidence to explain the last moments of 'Jumpin'' Johnny Montantes. Only now, months on, I don't mind. I prefer it this way, in fact. I've given up on ever seeing the full fight, or the knockout for a third time, and I no longer pester James about it, either.

For me to say this I know something has changed; some kind of lesson has been learnt. I got too close in Vegas, too keen, too involved. I understand that now. I might not have witnessed a tragedy in person but Crayton showing me how it all went down in the Mardi Gras ballroom, complete with action replays, was as close to being there, as close to witnessing another man perish, as one could ever wish to get: The Next Worst Thing.

For two of Crayton's seven children, sons James Jr, twenty-three, and Dominique, twenty-one, this moment of clarity, this realisation they had gone too deep, arrived three years ago. It, the moment, changed their view of their father and, pivotally, their outlook on boxing, a game – to them – which had up until that point piqued their curiosity. 'My twenty-one-year-old, in particular, said he wanted to continue my name in the sport, but he's not dedicated,' Crayton earlier explained to me. 'He's not in the gym like I was in the gym. I was in the gym every single day for four hours. My son doesn't do that. He drinks, he smokes.'

Whenever Dominique overstepped the mark and pestered his father about entering the fight game, Crayton brought out his trump card – Johnny Montantes. He would ask, 'Are you prepared to go to those lengths? Are you willing to take that risk?' Dominique, young, directionless and full of testosterone, would nod his head and puff out his chest, high on self-belief because he'd been taken to the gym a few times and been told he'd inherited his father's right hand. 'It's just decent,' Crayton said. 'I'm not going to say it's as good as mine.'

There's another reason James knows what he knows.

'Are you boys going to try me?' he asked James Jr and Dominique in the gym three years ago. 'You think you can take me now you're all grown up?'

James Jr, the older, more intuitive sibling, took a step back and shook his head. His dreams are now in the rap game. But Dominique, the one who has always fancied himself as a fighter, stood stoically and said nothing, much to his father's chagrin. His reaction stuck with James. It bugged him. *How dare my son think he can take me*, he thought.

Next time they went to the gym, James decided to test Dominique for real. See if he was truly as confident as he made out. 'Okay,' he said, 'today you're going to spar me.'

'Huh?' said Dominique.

'You. Are. Going. To. Spar. Me.'

Dominique laughed.

'You do you and I'll do me. Let's see what happens.'

'I won't hurt you, Dad.'

Crayton flashed a wry smile. 'You'll *never* hurt me, son.'

They went at it. Father stalked, son tried to escape. A body shot went in, thrown by father, absorbed by son, and a pained gasp was emitted from an open mouth. 'Are you okay?' asked the older man, the former pro. Dominique shrugged. He moved some more. He tried to jab, jab, jab. One was lazy, however, and his father instinctively countered over the top with a punch that dropped Dominique to the canvas.

He got up and the same nonchalant shrug followed. Only

now his face was serious, fearful even. His sphincter tightened. No longer was he half-heartedly sparring his dad, the man who brought him into this world. Now it was a proper fight. Now it was war. Life or death. They shared head space just as they shared a ring. Both wanted to hurt the other.

Loading up, father and son bit down and exchanged hard punches before a trademark James Crayton right hand, detonated for old times' sake by a forty-two-year-old with a message to send, landed flush on Dominique's chin and knocked him the fuck out.

Dominique woke moments later to a blurred image of his father standing over him. He was then pulled upright. 'I'm going to ask you a question,' said James, brushing his son down, 'and I won't get mad and I won't whup your butt.' He looked his offspring in the eyes. 'Remember I asked you and your brother if you guys were going to try me?'

Dominique meekly nodded his head.

'You didn't say anything. Did you think you'd whup my ass?'

'Yeah, Dad, I did,' said Dominique.

'And why did you think that?'

'Because you're getting older.'

'And what do you think now?'

'Naw, you've still got it.'

'Don't *ever* think you can whup me, man.'

Dominique, like me, got too close to something he could never truly understand.

THE DOG ROUNDS

ROUND ONE

1991: Straight down to it, they'd been here before. Chris Eubank came out back-peddling, threatening to explode with the odd, sudden, jarring right hand, and was once again the complete antithesis to Michael Watson in terms of style. Watson's style, guard held high, gloves cupped around the sides of his face like oversized ear muffs, seemed learned, textbook, whereas Eubank's seemed wholly improvised. He set traps. He worked on instinct, a feeling, a whim. He relied on athleticism. Watson prepared to counteract unpredictability as best he could. He stalked Eubank in round one and dug in body shots, lefts and rights, in an attempt to slow him down. Each time he did so there were cheers and chants from many among the 22,000 fans at White Hart Lane, home of Tottenham Hotspur Football Club. A peculiar thing, too, because Watson was an Arsenal fan, and had even worn their logo on his robe. Then again, this was a fight, not a football match, and in the context of a fight, any old fight, many wanted to see Chris Eubank bashed up and humbled. It was always the way.

2016: Chris Eubank Jr rarely starts proceedings the old-fashioned way, which is to say straight down to business, but he does so against Nick Blackwell, a sign perhaps of begrudging respect. Gone is the posing and posturing which has blighted some of his previous wins against overmatched Latvians and Lithuanians. This one, in contrast, feels like one of the few proper fights he has had. He flicks out the jab. He moves and samples, with his feet, every inch of the canvas. At times he scurries like his old man. When close, he bangs Blackwell to the body with right hands and then ties him up. Blackwell, eager to retaliate, is often too slow. He walks Eubank Jr down and throws out his stiff jab, but this one-dimensional approach gives Eubank Jr openings. An uppercut a minute and a half into the round, for example, jolts Blackwell's head and precipitates a call for the challenger to 'bring it on!' Blackwell drops his hands and invites more of the same. He will get his wish.

ROUND TWO

1991: The name of the game continued to be surprise as Eubank stood still to begin round two, momentarily frozen in time, and then ducked his head low and catapulted a rash right hand the way of Watson as soon as he encroached his territory. It failed. It had no impact. But the method was clear. Eubank believed he'd gain success in the bout from one shot. He had *that* much faith in his power. Watson, of course, disagreed. He went after Eubank even harder in the second and had him scuttling around the ring's perimeter. There was no evident fear of the power he possessed, nor was he a sucker for single shots. Flurries were different, mind. Eubank's flurries, when thrown, were able to penetrate Watson's guard and fluster him. He gained success this way in the early going. 'Break him down, Michael!' said a wise voice from his corner.

2016: Traps are being set. Eubank Jr retreats to a neutral corner, as he did in round one, and Blackwell pounces. He gets excited, he unloads punches, he knows the chances of catching Eubank Jr stationary are few and far between; right hands graze the back of the challenger's head and his shoulders. But Eubank Jr then shakes his head dismissively. He throws a left uppercut and right hand, which miss, before rattling off more rights into Blackwell's midsection. They appear to have no effect. Blackwell continues coming forward and throwing out his jab. He's timing it better now, too. One knocks Eubank Jr off balance as he tries to mimic his father with a reckless right, while another puts him back on his heels. It reminds Eubank Jr to sharpen up. He does so in the form of a right and left to the body followed by a beautifully picked right uppercut, a sign once again he possesses the variety.

ROUND THREE

1991: Wavelengths and bodies connected in round three as both Eubank and Watson met in the centre of the ring and *immediately* started throwing. There was no let-up. Eubank still pursued a home for his sneaky right hand, while Watson, far from smooth, having had to switch from natural counter-puncher to makeshift aggressor, tried to force the pace and, at times, wasted energy in doing so. Still, a right hand thrown as Eubank prepped his own definitely registered, as did the chopping right Watson rained down on his opponent as he ducked for cover. Referee Roy Francis split them from a clinch and Eubank spat on the canvas. It was a sign things were heating up, that it was time to get down and dirty. They swung rights at the same time. Both landed. Eubank dipped to avoid the follow-up, then seemed content to hold.

2016: In an odd turn of events, it's Blackwell doing the Eubank act to start round three. He pouts and poses in anticipation of the bell, as if having studied his opponent's father, and then gallops towards the middle of the ring behind his high-held guard. Soon he gets Eubank Jr where he wants him, which is trapped on the ropes, but finds himself still out-landed when the challenger emerges with combinations and countless uppercuts. One right uppercut lands and ignites something in Blackwell. He trades back. The crowd get to their feet. They sense something special. They celebrate violence. Blackwell, though, calms down and returns to his jab. All in good time, he seems to say. He pops a jab in the face of Eubank Jr, a shot well-timed, and this again knocks him off balance. Eubank Jr shakes it off. He wiggles his hips. The crowd of around 2,500 mock him. In answer, he uncorks another blindingly fast combination, including a left hook so startling it has Blackwell momentarily feeling like he's surrounded. Regardless, he begs for more.

ROUND FOUR
1991: To start round four Eubank threw a right hand so unorthodox and circular in its motion it seemed he was

winding up to hit a high striker at a fairground. Everything went into it. All his might. He wanted top score. But, still, it had no impact. Watson smothered it as he rolled forward and was quick to sink a left uppercut into his rival's belly, a punch ruled 'low' by the referee. Aiming back at the head, both churned out crosses at mid-range, some landing, some missing, and Eubank was soon cut over his left eye – a small nick above the eyelid – as well as on the run. 'What a fight,' said ITV commentator Reg Gutteridge to close out the round.

2016: Rat-a-tat-tat goes the jab of Eubank Jr as he skates around the ring and uses that particular punch to befuddle Blackwell and create openings. It's an effective ploy, too, because off the jab, consecutive right uppercuts land flush and knock the champion's head back. Eubank Jr then capitalises on this momentum and goes after Blackwell, turning the tables, driving him to the ropes. More punches are uncoiled. Blackwell answers with a right of his own and Eubank Jr decides to back off with his hands by his sides. He smiles, consults his jab. Moments later, he will reveal another trap, this time retreating to the corner of his own volition and goading Blackwell. He then makes Blackwell miss and they swap hooks in close. After that, Eubank Jr goes for a walk and buys some time. He tours the ring. Blackwell's nose and mouth are covered in blood. He grimaces, the taste on his tongue.

ROUND FIVE

1991: Watson now brought more than just pressure and pace. He was landing clean shots as well. Two rights, for instance, thrown one after the other, caught Eubank and sent him to the ropes. He then looked to land more. Eubank, to his credit, remained composed, unflappable. Nothing changed the expression on his face when punches were exchanged. He simply moved, created space and then pot-shotted rights of his own whenever the opportunity presented itself. He may have been getting outworked, and desperate for a lull in the action, but still he placed belief in his ability to turn things around with one punch. Just one. Nigel Benn, sat ringside, hoped that wouldn't be the case. He told ITV's Gary Newbon in between rounds, 'Nobody deserves to win a title more than Michael [Watson].'

2016: Blackwell catches Eubank Jr with a right hand and follows with three more, thrown as Eubank Jr sneaks low and tries to hold. They scuff the top of his head. Eubank Jr, once upright, lands some more body shots and then back-to-back right uppercuts which give Blackwell whiplash. Richie Woodhall, Channel 5's co-commentator, worries Blackwell might be taking too many. He says he needs to get to the later rounds, his territory, but to ideally take less punishment in the process. As if hearing this, Blackwell ups his urgency, pins Eubank Jr in a neutral corner and throws everything he has. Eubank Jr, though, trembles like a man being tasered, making himself almost impossible to hit, and then gets away with the help of a clinch. Once free, he proceeds to overwhelm Blackwell with punches, shoving him towards the corner, and even gestures to someone at ringside with his left glove before launching that same glove the way of his opponent. It looks good but it's blocked. Not only that, a lapse in concentration has emerged. Lo and behold, as Eubank Jr continues to throw hands haphazardly, Blackwell connects with a right counter, his best shot of the fight, and it wobbles the cocky challenger. The crowd erupt. They think he's hurt. But a wry smile, flashed moments after returning his gum shield to his mouth, reveals that's not the case.

ROUND SIX

1991: Eubank pushed Watson towards the canvas with his right glove and then motioned for him to rise. No time for respite. The referee, however, admonished Eubank for pushing, told the timekeeper it wasn't a knockdown and then wiped Watson's gloves before signalling the restart. On command, they went at it again. Eubank auditioned some more Hail Mary right hands, his supposed pay-off punch, while Watson methodically marched him down, caught him in corners and tried to stop him squirming away. Both had success. Watson would sometimes get a little too keen in exchanges and leave himself open to Eubank counters, but Eubank, also, seemed to be tiring in this round and appeared impatient for the bell. Of course, when it finally sounded, he stood on the spot, tapped his gloves together and convinced all he was in complete control. He was Chris Eubank, after all.

2016: Buoyed by the right hand he landed in the previous round, Blackwell strides forward with renewed vigour in the sixth. He chops down more rights whenever he gets Eubank Jr close. He tries to rough him up. He follows him diligently and to such an extent that Gary Lockett, his trainer, signals for him to cut off the ring by taking a big step to his right. But still Blackwell continues to aimlessly follow. It works for Eubank Jr. He keeps dictating the play, peppering Blackwell with his jab, and then glides forward behind his left shoulder, used to protect his chin from harm, whenever he wants to rest in a clinch. Once comfortable in this position, he slots in uppercut after uppercut, snapping Blackwell's head back like a speedball. Not once does Blackwell appear hurt, however; through a bloody mask, he sticks out his tongue and outwardly relishes the onslaught.

ROUND SEVEN

1991: The more Eubank tried to move, the more Watson made a concentrated effort to target his body with hooks and uppercuts. It was a simple plan. It was, Watson believed, a method of slowing him down and creating openings upstairs. This proved the case in round seven. Body shots paved the way for a left hook and two right crosses, which nailed a stationary Eubank. Suddenly he looked disorganised again. Right hands were aimed over his low left hand and he was being ambushed. 'Keep your hands up, Mike,' came a shout from Watson's corner. They sensed he was winning, that the momentum was with him, but they also knew how quickly it could all change.

2016: Eubank Jr comes out blasting. Thirty seconds in, he lands uppercuts at will, turns them into hooks and then, with Blackwell against the ropes, drills shots to his body. Blackwell throws back, of course, if only to show he's not hurt, but this just leaves him open to more of the same. Uppercuts smash into his already bloody nose, double and triple left hook combinations highlight the difference in speed, and Gary Lockett, Blackwell's third eye, peers through the ropes, a look of concern on his face, to make sure his man is okay. He is. Just about. One right hand thrown in response gets him out of trouble and creates space. But Eubank Jr is now relentless. He traps Blackwell on the other side of the ring and rattles through his extensive arsenal of punches all over again. Blood covers the lower half of Blackwell's face. He swallows three uppercuts in close and keeps pressing forward. 'Do you like taking these uppercuts, or what?' Lockett asks his fighter in the corner.

ROUND EIGHT

1991: 'By now Eubank should be trying to hurt Watson,' said ITV co-commentator Jim Watt. 'Stand his ground, use his strength, and use his punching power... but he's still being backed up and he hasn't really tried to stop Watson in his tracks. I think it's high time he did that.' There were certainly opportunities for him. Both men were tiring at this stage, their work had become sloppy, and such was Watson's exuberance, he often left openings. Eubank exploited this on occasion. He timed Watson's swings and punched in between them. A right hand, in particular, seemed to have an impact in round eight. It made Watson stop and think, if only for a moment. But, once his head cleared, he was back on Eubank, working both hands, desperate to win the round, unwilling to allow his rival to have the final say in any exchange.

2016: Chris Eubank, the father, now forty-nine, lingers a little too long between rounds and is told off by referee Victor Loughlin. 'Seconds out' means exactly that. Get out the ring. He does as he's told, albeit belatedly, and the round starts. Richie Woodhall, in commentary, calls for Blackwell to employ a cross-armed defence (forearms positioned horizontally in front of face) against the Eubank Jr uppercut. He says it would serve him well. Blackwell is oblivious to such advice, though. Besides, it's not solely the uppercuts causing him problems. Four left hooks, for example, whack him around the head and back him into a neutral corner, before Eubank Jr then throws every other possible shot his way, including a series of manic left and right hooks, all dispatched with a deranged look on his face. Blackwell offers a right hand of his own to show his survival instincts are still intact, but Eubank Jr can't understand how or why the fight continues. He looks out at the crowd, shrugs, and points at Blackwell as if to say, 'How is he still in this?' They then grin at each other. Blackwell, unconcerned, pushes Eubank Jr into a corner and tries to hit something, *anything*, but his work noticeably lacks the snap and power of his counterpart. They end up in a tired embrace. Eubank Jr takes a deep breath as he returns to his corner. Specks of Blackwell's blood cover his back and shoulders.

'If the referee doesn't stop it, I don't know what to tell you,' Chris Eubank says to his son as they convene in the corner. 'If he doesn't stop it, and you keep on beating him like this, one, he's getting hurt, and, two, if it goes to a decision, why hasn't the referee stopped the fight? I don't know why. So maybe you shouldn't leave it to the referee. But you're not going to take him out to the face, you're going to take him out to the body. Okay?'

Ronnie Davies spreads Vaseline around the boxer's face, then adds, 'Do it your way. Okay, mate? Your way's working.'

ROUND NINE

1991: There was more scurrying from Eubank to start round nine. There were more crazy right hands as well, first thrown as wide hooks, then shortened in the form of an uppercut which grabbed Watson's attention. But still it was Watson who demonstrated the consistency and better technique. He landed a jab and right hand clean on Eubank as he tried to move along the ropes and the crowd immediately showed their appreciation. They, like Watson, believed Eubank was folding. 'Watson just seems to disregard the punches Eubank lands on him,' said Watt. 'He's totally fired up.'

2016: The pace drops. Both are content to trade jabs. Eubank Jr shoots high and low, stabbing the punches towards Blackwell's midsection, while Blackwell tries in vain to land his right over Eubank Jr's sometimes sloppy left hand. Is Eubank Jr acting on his father's instructions? Well, if not yet a pacifist, he has certainly reined himself in. He now just pops the jab. There's not much purpose or power behind it; it touches Blackwell and the large swelling above his left eye from afar. The uppercuts and hooks have also dried up, though perhaps this owes to tiredness.

'He's knackered, he's on the back foot, but you're not putting him under pressure,' Lockett tells Blackwell in the corner. 'You've got to start doing it if you want to win this fight. Literally all the snap has gone out of his punches. This was the plan to take him now. The kid's feet have slowed, his jab has slowed, his punches have slowed. He's reluctant now to tee off. This is where you've got to come out and dig in. This is what you've wanted your whole life, isn't it? We've been thinking about this fight for a year. We knew you weren't going to beat him on the outside, so you need to get closer and work him over, twos and threes.'

While this goes on, Bob Plant, the cuts man, wipes the blood from Blackwell's face and puts two swabs up his nostrils. He then applies Vaseline to his deformed brow.

ROUND TEN

1991: Two Watson right hands knocked Eubank off balance and he immediately covered up. Yet, from that very position, that shell, he still managed to spit a counter left hook which caught Watson rising from a crouch. Now it was on. Watson, both annoyed and energised, nailed Eubank with a short right at centre ring and it stopped Eubank in his tracks. He swayed towards the ropes, either hurt or pretending he was hurt, and cleverly made Watson miss his follow-up assault. Arms by his sides, Eubank remained a picture of hubris and liked to believe he was in control. The swelling by his left eye, though, said otherwise.

2016: Acting on Lockett's pick-me-up, Blackwell hurries to the centre of the ring to begin round ten. He's greeted there by Eubank Jr, who punches him to the body, then punctures his guard with scything uppercuts, a fixture of the contest. Blackwell backs up to the ropes. The pressure continues. Eubank Jr is well in control, but Blackwell has still to show any obvious signs of being hurt. *Properly hurt*. He has not, as far as the eye can see, been shaken, dazed or even buzzed. His posture remains sturdy. His left eye, though, is fast closing. There are concerned faces at ringside. The referee, Victor Loughlin, gets close and then, as Eubank Jr drops his hands to his sides and offers Blackwell free shots at his unguarded face, makes his move. He uses the lull in the action as an opportunity to call 'time' and take Blackwell towards the ringside doctor. 'Come here, doctor,' he says. People start to boo. The doctor climbs up on the ring apron, whispers into the referee's ear and the fight is waved off two minutes and twenty-one seconds into round ten. It wasn't the conclusive finish he wanted, but Eubank Jr takes it. He climbs a ring post and laps up the acclaim. 'Blackwell will fight on, of course, and has much in front of him, but Eubank Jr was too tough and too good for him here tonight,' is the assessment of

Channel 5 commentator Dave Farrar. 'Whatever the method of the result, it's the right result.'

ROUND ELEVEN

1991: At long last Eubank found some distance, some breathing room, and cracked Watson with a good right hand. It was accompanied by a left, a right and another left as if he were in a pool performing the front crawl. Watson placed his left hand over Eubank's right shoulder and locked him in a clinch. It was safer there. But Eubank, once separated, wouldn't let up. He put Watson back in a defensive posture, up against the ropes, and pulled the trigger on more wayward rights. It then got messy as slack ring ropes nearly resulted in both boxers tumbling out of the ring in the middle of an exchange. 'The ropes are far too slack,' said Gutteridge.

On they went, however. Watson tagged Eubank inside with short shots, forced him to cover up, and then landed a hook which buzzed him, followed by an uppercut, a cuffing right and a huge left–right combination, which shut down Eubank as he attempted to respond. The final two shots did the damage. They took it all out of Eubank. Zombified him. He had no option but to fall to his knees, an act which signified the first clean knockdown of his professional career, with sixteen seconds left in the round. Watson was on the verge. He knew it now. So too did Eubank, who sprung to his feet immediately, too proud to take the full count (as it happened, a count waived by referee Francis, so surprised was he to find Eubank on the deck).

At the restart, with a buoyant Watson lodged in a neutral corner, Eubank stepped to the centre of the ring, loaded his right hand and blindly let the uppercut go. It was thrown as though it was the last punch he would ever throw. He later claimed it contained 'frustration, exhaustion, resolve and instinct'. Whatever the ingredients, it found Watson's chin, just as he was positioning his hands in his defensive cocoon, and sent him flying to the canvas on his backside, his neck snapping against the second rope. With that, the course of the fight was changed. Lives were changed. Watson rose as quickly as he could, a mark of the man's doughtiness and determination, but he was never the same again. Jimmy Tibbs, his coach, had to scamper after him to bring him back to the stool. 'An absolutely sensational eleventh round,' remarked Gutteridge and everyone else.

2016: After being consoled by near-enough every member of the Eubank family, Blackwell stands and listens to his fate read back to him by the master of ceremonies. He soon won't remember this moment or, indeed, anything else about the fight, but is told he has been stopped on the advice of the ringside doctor. He then watches Eubank Jr, the victor, pose with the British title he once wore.

On any other day, all this would hurt. *Really* hurt. But Blackwell, a vacant look on his face, no longer feels his normal self. He tells Gary Lockett he is dizzy and weak. He stumbles on the way back to his corner. He's sat down on his stool. He's administered oxygen. He loses consciousness. He'll soon leave the ring on a stretcher.

Helpless as the rest of them, I watch this scene unfold from my position at ringside and crudely mutter to a stranger, an Irishman, stood beside me, 'This is fucking awful.' I mean the situation, the cruel, unfair nature of it. I also mean boxing.

ROUND TWELVE
1991: Eubank rose from his stool first, which, given the events of the previous round, was no great surprise. When Watson

eventually emerged, however, he seemed rooted to the spot, his legs unable to carry him towards the middle of the ring, and the referee had to grab his left arm and pull him forward in order for him to touch gloves with Eubank before the final round, as per the etiquette of the sport. From there, Watson retreated to a neutral corner and Eubank immediately knew he was finished, gone. He wound up a hook and followed its trajectory into Watson, throwing both hands along the way. Francis separated them as they fell into a clinch, but Watson stayed put. He moved barely an inch. This allowed Eubank another chance to hit him and keep hitting him. He landed two consecutive right hands, which sent Watson's head up in the air, and that was enough to force Francis to do the right thing and end the contest just twenty-nine seconds into the last round.

Eubank raised both arms in celebration. He would soon discover Watson was ahead on all three judges' scorecards at the time of the stoppage. Not that he needed to be told. He *felt* it. 'It wasn't the damage Eubank inflicted in the last round,' said Watt. 'The damage was done in the previous round – that one shot.'

The extent of the damage became clear to all once some petty skirmishes in the crowd had been dispersed, interviews were concluded and Michael Watson was spotted lying down in his corner, unconscious, with his head resting on a doctor's briefcase. It was 10:56p.m. and the fighter had collapsed. Twelve minutes later, he was on a stretcher, had a tube in his mouth to aid his breathing (there was no emergency resuscitation equipment available at ringside), and was taken on an ill-timed tour of the venue before finding the waiting ambulance.

2016: It's the not knowing. That's the worst part. We don't know where Nick Blackwell has been taken, we don't know the severity of the damage and we don't know the ending.

I try looking for answers. His changing room is the obvious first port of call and I make a beeline for it minutes after the fight ends. By this time, the stricken boxer has been hurried out the venue and loaded into an ambulance. I know that much. But the debris left behind is as revealing as any prognosis. Friends, family and trainers are strewn across the changing-room floor, some on their hands and knees, others alone in each of the four corners, and only the ones still able to function, the ones capable of putting one foot in front of the other, gather up their gear and follow the ambulance to the designated hospital. For the rest, it is too much.

I have nothing to say to any of them. I hug Nick's best friend Jake, for it seems the only human thing to do in the moment, but that is it. No words fall from my mouth. All I can do is stand at the entrance of the changing room, watching, sympathising, wondering.

Soon enough, the room is empty. *That* room. The same room in which Blackwell had earlier wrapped his hands, smiled, cracked jokes, warmed up, gloved up, stretched, shadowboxed, hit pads and readied his body and mind for war. He got that at least. War. He played his part in that. But this wasn't the way it was supposed to end. He should have been back here by eleven o'clock, soaking up words of encouragement from family and friends, those so humbled by his courage, and he should have been nipping to the bathroom to try and summon enough piss, while in a state of extreme dehydration, to satisfy the official conducting the post-fight drug test. *That* was the process. Not this.

THE DOG ROUNDS

ROUND THIRTEEN

1991: It was 11:22p.m. when Watson, pupils fixed and dilated (a sign his brain stem had suffered an injury), arrived at the North Middlesex hospital. It was also the wrong place; there was inadequate resuscitation equipment and no specialist head trauma staff (since the Eubank–Watson II fight, regulations stipulate that there has to be a neurological hospital within ten minutes of the arena in which a professional boxing event takes place). Watson's brain had been starved of oxygen for thirty minutes. He'd suffered an acute subdural haemorrhage, a blood clot on the surface of the brain, an injury caused in round eleven by the impact of Chris Eubank's right uppercut and the impact of his head then hitting the ropes, and was rushed from North Middlesex to St Bartholomew's Hospital by 11:55p.m., one minute outside the so-called 'golden hour' all neurosurgeons hold so dear.

A call was made to Dr Peter Hamlyn, Barts' consultant neurosurgeon, shortly after Watson arrived and had been assessed. Hamlyn, enjoying a day off from surgery, jumped in a taxi and raced to the hospital, but was unable to enter due to the sheer number of people outside wanting to gawp or gain information. Up against the clock, he directed his taxi to the back of the building, searched for an open door and made it inside as Watson was prepared for surgery.

This would be Hamlyn's third operation on a boxer. The other two boxers survived. But, crucial to this particular case, some two hours had passed from the moment of Watson's collapse to the start of surgery and Hamlyn, because of this, would one day admit, 'Michael was closer to death than anybody I have ever operated on.'

2016: Some things continue. The requirement for reporters to speak to the victor, for example, is one that continues in spite of the general malaise and uncertainty surrounding the ex-champion. Mike Legg of the *Argus*, Chris Eubank Jr's local newspaper, collars me as I wander cluelessly around the arena and requests I take him backstage to check in with the winner and his father. So that's what we do.

This time the changing room is full. Nobody sheds a tear. These are happier faces for the most part; they are the faces of satisfaction, pleased their boy, Chris Eubank Jr, has won the British middleweight title, pleased he's heading home relatively unscathed. But then there is Ronnie Davies, the boy's trainer, who seems significantly less happy than the others; arms crossed, face creased by a permanent frown, he sits on a chair by the entrance to the room and shakes his head as if it is the only motion permitted.

We ask him what is wrong.

'His [Blackwell's] corner should have pulled him out of there or the referee should have stopped it,' snaps Ronnie, who offered his own towel for Blackwell to use as a 'pillow' once horizontal. 'That boy took way too much punishment. I knew he'd be too brave for his own good and he was. He took a bad beating, nobody thought to stop it and now he's in hospital.'

'When, in your opinion, should it have been stopped?' I ask.

'I thought he should have been stopped around the seventh. He was just getting beaten up. He was getting thrashed. It was a severe beating. I thought Eubank was unbelievable, I thought he was great, but I don't feel happy right now.'

Given how infuriated Davies appears, I reconsider my own

thoughts on the fight. Was it truly as one-sided as he claimed? Was it as severe a beating as he had us believe? Should it have been stopped earlier? None of these ideas were even in my head before I ventured into the Eubank changing room. But now I can't shake them. In light of this, was I the masochist? Was I the one who had become desensitised by violence, by this sport, to such an extent that I failed to realise a boxer I respected and liked was being badly dominated and hurt? Davies, in the heat of the moment, makes it sound ghastly. He makes us all out to be monsters. Nobody escapes his pointing finger.

Chris Eubank, on the other hand, is more considered in his approach. He paces the room in a contemplative state, suited and booted, sans cane, and picks carefully from a plastic container of pineapple slices. Only when he is ready to talk does he talk.

'I am immensely proud of his performance,' he says, pointing towards the bathroom door (Eubank Jr is trying to produce a urine sample for the post-fight drug test). 'We're British champions and it's something we're very proud of. He has quenched the thirst. I didn't want him in my shadow because I knew he was better than that. But he needed to prove it. He did that tonight. Maybe now they'll start hearing what I said the other day at the press conference. Junior is a very dangerous man. The referees have to look after the opponents.'

He is asked if he, like Davies, believes the fight should have been stopped earlier.

'It was madness,' he says. 'Two rounds before it was stopped he hit him with a flurry of punches and I'm like, "What's going on?" I banged on the ring canvas and at the end of the round the referee said, "Do not bang on the canvas!" He told me not to tell him how to do his job.'

Eubank mimics the zipping of his mouth. He then allows it to open again to engulf an incoming pineapple slice. As he chews, the local reporter pounces. He asks him if he feared the worst. 'You could see it,' goes the reply. 'He was like, "Bring it." But he was too tough for his own good. That's why I said to you,' he now points at me, 'you have to protect these guys. You have to protect them from themselves. He was getting hit and was like, "Is that all you've got? Bring it, bring it, bring it." We don't do that. No macho stuff.'

Inevitably, Michael Watson is in the air.

'You can see I'm teary now, can't you?' says Eubank.

It was no lie. His eyes, watery, look directly at me and he clenches his jaw in a manner which suggests it is the only way of stopping his face from crumbling.

'You've been there,' I say.

'It's not that I've been there. I *am* there. That obsession has not left me. I'm still obsessed. I'm living with this. I know this life. I said to Nick Blackwell the other day, "This is not a game." To spectators it's a game, but to us it's a way of life. People lose their lives in this sport. Is it a mug's game?'

'It was a mug's game tonight,' Davies laments from his chair in the corner.

'We're real, we're fierce, we're not jokers,' Senior emphasises. 'Junior has a type of cold where he'll say, "It's just part of the game."'

As if eavesdropping, Chris Junior suddenly appears. The bathroom door opens slightly and his head pops through the gap created. There is no smile, no projection of pride. He merely requests a towel, immediately thrown to him by one of his friends, and then vanishes again.

THE DOG ROUNDS

ROUND FOURTEEN

1991: The surgery to remove a clot the size of a saucer of milk from the left side of Michael Watson's brain and stem a subdural haemorrhage, the first of six procedures, was over by 4:20a.m., but the prognosis remained ominous. Watson was placed in intensive care, where he was visited by first his mother Joan, and then, at 5:10a.m., by his trainer, Jimmy Tibbs.

Chris Eubank, meanwhile, was physically and emotionally spent and could hardly stand, let alone move. He returned to his changing room after the fight to be told Watson was hurt, but wouldn't know just how hurt until he later saw him at the hospital. It was then, after his own treatment for exhaustion and internal injuries, that he visited his former opponent at around 1:30a.m. The sight that greeted him was horrifying. Watson was in a coma with a quarter of his skull missing. 'My very soul shuddered,' Eubank would say.

2016: 'I don't know if you could hear me between rounds,' Chris Eubank continues, still picking pineapple from a plastic pot. 'What did I say to him, Ron? I said, "Take it easy on him. Leave his face alone. Punch his body. You don't need to hit him in the head any more. The fight is yours." He said, "No. I want to teach him a lesson."'

The father shrugs as if to say, 'What could I do?'

The video of father instructing son to throw punches to the body instead of the head will soon take the internet by storm; a sign of post-Watson compassion provoking a need to protect Blackwell to some, it is deemed merely a tactical call in the eyes of many who follow the sport. But, now, minutes after the fight has ended, Eubank has no idea the moment was even captured on film, much less realises it will prove so ambiguous and open to interpretation. None of us do. So, before he has a chance to perhaps rewrite history and prepare his answer, thus anointing himself The Knight in Shiny Winklepickers, I ask him, 'Why did you say that?'

'I'm not like Junior,' he says. 'Junior is cold. He's ruthless. But that's what the British public will appreciate about him. They want to see an annihilation. They want to see a man eviscerated. Junior will be only too happy to oblige. The British public want that in a British champion. This is boxing. What he is, I can't put my finger on it. But it isn't reasonable.'

'The uppercuts were landing over and over again,' says Ronnie Davies, still arguing with no one and everyone. 'I feel so sorry for that kid. This wasn't a one shot thing like he [Eubank] did against Watson. This was a sustained beating. There were chances to stop it and they weren't taken. A severe beating like this was worse than the one shot he caught Watson with. Innit, Chris?'

'Absolutely. It should have been stopped. We know Junior. People say he doesn't punch hard, that he punches in bunches, but he *does* punch hard. They are concussive punches.'

Davies continues shaking his head. 'His career is finished,' he says. 'No matter what happens now, that kid will not fight again. He took too much punishment and is probably damaged now.'

Senior looks to the floor. His container of pineapple is now empty. He starts on a box of coconut slices instead. 'That was a damaging fight,' he muses, prising the box open. 'A *very* damaging fight.'

'He came straight forward in a line,' says Davies. 'Anyone who wants to come and fight Eubank has fucking had it.

I don't care what weight they are. I feel sorry for them. I feel deeply upset for that kid. I feel deeply upset that he's going to hospital and none of us know whether he's going to make it or not. Why does a kid have to take punishment unnecessarily? I've been in this game all my life and I can't remember a beating like that. When did you last see a beating like that, Chris?'

Eubank shrugs. 'I haven't seen a beating like that since the forties,' he says.

'That's right. You go back to fights with guys like Jake LaMotta...'

Eubank Jr re-emerges from the bathroom, causes an immediate hush, and locates a can of Lynx chocolate deodorant which he uses to spray his armpits. While doing so he asks about the scoring of the fight – how the judges had it, how television had it – and then shakes his head upon hearing Channel 5, the night's broadcasters, only had him four rounds up at the time of the stoppage. Not that it matters. Not that anything matters now.

Within thirteen and a half minutes of leaving the ring, Nick Blackwell is placed in an induced coma while in the back of an ambulance en route to St Mary's Hospital in Paddington. Not long after that, his body shuts down, he flatlines, and his name becomes the latest addition to a never-ending, unholy list of ring casualties. Before even reaching the hospital, he dies.

'I've accomplished the task,' says Eubank Jr. 'I can look back on my legacy and say, "I became British champion." It was a hell of a fight. I'm very proud.'

He is asked if he thought the fight should have been stopped.

'The warrior in me wanted the fight to continue,' he says.

'The warrior wants to finish the fight in exciting fashion. I was going to go out there and search and destroy, as I did in the sixth and a few of the other rounds, and the referee would have had to jump in or he would have been knocked out. The referee should have stopped the fight way before then.'

Okay, enough. His father abruptly holds out his hand, clouding the daylight between reporter and subject, and then turns it into a single index finger. 'Hold on,' he says. 'We don't know the outcome of what has happened. I think we have to wait and see how Nick is. Everything he says and you print, depending on how he comes out of this, could be deemed insensitive. As he said, he's very happy to be British champion, but that's as much as he can give you. Let's see what happens. Words like "warrior" and "search and destroy" you have to go easy on, because we don't know Nick's state. People will think he said it after he knew his state. We're not doing that.'

It is one intrusion, one interruption, that makes absolute sense. Timed to perfection, it is a protective and compassionate move, one perhaps only a former fighter would make.

'Nick *is* a warrior,' Junior continues, getting dressed. 'He earned that title tonight. Someone taking that punishment for that many rounds and not giving up, it's admirable. That's how fighters should be. We go out on our shield. We have that mentality. Don't give up until the referee stops it. He's a solid guy and he had a lot of grit and determination. I have a lot of respect for him.'

Around this time a shot of adrenalin, injected directly into Nick Blackwell's heart, brings a warrior back to life.

THE DOG ROUNDS

ROUND FIFTEEN

1991: Watson spent a total of forty days in a coma and brain damage left him paralysed with no control over his body. For a while, once on the road to recovery, the only way he could communicate was through blinking his eyes or moving his fingers to indicate 'yes' or 'no'. He was completely immobile, he couldn't move his hands or legs, and he couldn't hold his head up. He dribbled. He had to be fed through a straw; to swallow, his jaw had to be rubbed by a carer. More or less a prisoner in his own body, details of Watson's condition 'shredded' Chris Eubank.

But, after nearly two years of intensive physio and speech therapy, 'The People's Champion' finally went home.

2016: Three days later, on the Tuesday, the Eubanks hold a press conference at the Jumeirah Carlton Tower in Sloane Street, Knightsbridge, the supposed purpose of which is to address the nation's media, the majority of whom didn't show any interest in the weekend's British middleweight title fight until it became a news story, and to talk about Junior's future. But, upon getting wind of the idea, Blackwell's family and his promoter, Mick Hennessy, beg the Eubanks, via a number of text messages sent from St Mary's Hospital, to postpone. They say it is in 'bad taste' and 'too soon'. Chris Eubank, however, assures them the press conference will be handled with sensitivity and that the main focus will be on his son's plans going forward. So, in spite of the Blackwell family's wishes, it goes ahead.

With a Union Jack flag draped across the table, and the British championship belt also present, Eubank tells those in attendance that his family will not celebrate the victory until they know Nick Blackwell has made a full recovery (three days on, he remains in an induced coma). He then goes on to explain that even in sparring he often implores his son to avoid hitting partners in the head and to instead target the body (this was in response to claims he had done the same in the Blackwell fight). 'In his last sparring session, I said, "No head shots,"' Eubank begins. '"If you don't watch your head shots, I'll stop the sparring." He [Junior] was very edgy because he was six days from the fight. He said, "You're not stopping my sparring." He's a stallion. You can't control him. I said to him, "I'm not going to test you, but don't test me. Don't test me!" I understand what happens with the shots. They take their toll. We are not fans of anyone who takes shots. There's nothing enlightening about being able to absorb great punishment. Yes, it shows great heart, but you must have the ability to actually protect your heart. The ability is gained by knowing the craft, which means you've got to be in the gym and treat it like a church. You have to go there and worship and learn this craft so you can protect your heart and keep on going. Nick's performance was magnificent in terms of his heart, but he didn't have the ability to protect his heart.'

'When I heard the news [of Blackwell's coma], it was tough,' says Chris Eubank Jr. 'We don't go in there to cause that type of damage to an opponent. Things are said, there's a lot of back and forth, and there's a lot of testosterone flying around, but no fighter wants to see their opponent in any type of serious condition. It was upsetting.

'It is business, not personal. I'm not going in there to ruin somebody's career and damage them. I just wanted to achieve my lifelong ambition of becoming British champion. It's a shame this has kind of taken away from it a little bit. But this is boxing. It's not a game. You play football, you play rugby, you play cricket. You don't play boxing. It's two men going in there and putting their lives on the line. It's not to be taken lightly.'

Oh, yes, Junior's future. As promised, this is touched upon, briefly, but only ever in the context of the Nick Blackwell situation. You know, how will he now respond? Will he view boxing differently? Will he find it difficult to continue? There is no talk of world titles or prospective opponents. They, the mainstream media, aren't here for that. Their interest in a boxer or, indeed, boxing, only reveals itself when all is dirty and dark, and is only ever fleeting.

'Not at all,' says Eubank Jr when asked if he'd find it tough to carry on. 'As fighters, we know the risks. We know we are risking our health every time we step into the ring. It's a risk we are willing to take because we know that with these risks come great reward. I've been boxing since I was fifteen years old. You hear the stories. You read up on them. Some [boxers] end up punch-drunk, some end up with serious injuries. You can't go into a fight worrying about that. If you go into a fight thinking you might get hurt, you most likely will. You need to go in there believing you are untouchable.'

His father is, of course, quick to elaborate. 'I lost my finishing instinct after that particular fight [Michael Watson], but that is not something I'm going to encourage,' he says. 'I'm going to steer him away from that. He has to be as ruthless as he can be. You cannot afford to have this sensitive mindset. He is in equal danger. The best way to protect him as a manager, as a father, as a mentor, is to tell him to keep the mindset he has, which is a warrior's mindset.'

'My goal is to become a world champion,' says Junior. 'I'm never going to realise that dream if I have any doubts or reservations about what happened to Nick. It may be cold but it's what we, as fighters, have to be. We have to have a certain coldness to do what we do. What has happened is a tragedy, but I can't let that stop me from fulfilling my dreams.'

Junior is asked, at one stage, if he ever felt concerned for his opposite number, a bizarre notion for any boxer to comprehend in the heat of battle.

'Nick was a warrior,' he says. 'He kept coming forward. He was even smiling when I hit him. He still had fight in him. Some people have said he was too tough for his own good but that's what you have to be as a fighter. You have to have that mentality. I don't care what you do to me, I don't care what you hit me with, or how much pain I'm in, I'm not stopping. I'm in there, in a fight, and Nick is trying to punch me in the face. You can't ask me if I was worried about him while I was fighting him. It's tough. When I'm watching him after the fight and he's lying on the ground with an oxygen mask on his face, that's when worry sets in. You think, wow, I didn't realise this was going to happen. I hope he's okay. I went over and said, "You're going to be all right, Nick. Everything will be okay." I think he was unconscious at the time. This is the sport. These things happen. It's never intentional.'

Ronnie Davies only clears his throat to say one thing, but, on reflection, it is perhaps the most revealing of all. 'I was very emotional [on the night],' he says. 'I've been through it with Chris. So, when I got back to the dressing room, I was deeply upset. I said the referee should have stopped it and his corner should have pulled him out.

'Looking back, though, thinking about it, watching the fight again, they couldn't. That kid was always there. He kept fighting back. And he's got a name for toughness. If you'd have pulled that kid out, it would have broke his heart. You couldn't pull the kid out. It's a title fight. It's his life.

'Now I think the referee and corner were right. I wish he hadn't kept fighting back. I wish he had gone down. It would have been easier. But he didn't. So what can you do? I didn't mean to disrespect the referee or his corner.'

What, I think, Ronnie Davies later came to realise, and what made Nick Blackwell's situation so wrong, is that everyone involved seemed to do everything right. The boxers, the trainers, the referee, the doctors, the paramedics, they all acted as they were supposed to act. This wasn't a weight-drained boxer beaten to a pulp against the ropes in full view of a negligent referee and corner team. This wasn't a boxer disposed to being knocked out succumbing to one too many within a short space of time. This wasn't a boxer with a prior brain condition that had slipped through the net. This one wasn't easily explainable.

Therefore, it could only be boxing and its sometimes glorious but sometimes heartless nature that was to blame.

14

THE RECOVERY

A sudden burst of sunlight brightens the room, emphasises his yellow complexion and highlights the damage a man's fists have done to his swollen face. It is Thursday, so five days after the fight, and Nick Blackwell is in St Mary's adult intensive care unit, all the way up on the ninth floor. He remains in an induced coma. There are tubes running from a respiratory machine to his mouth. His eyes are closed. His chest moves up and down at a rapid rate. The haematoma above his left eye, which had debilitated his vision on Saturday night, has now significantly reduced in size, and so too have other blemishes around his face, but still he wears the mask of a prizefighter: been in the wars, my grandmother would observe.

'Nick, if only you could see the sun right now,' says his promoter, Mick Hennessy, stood to the right of him. 'The sun's out, it's beautiful, it's great surfing weather. Come on, mate. We're supposed to meet you in Cornwall this summer.'

For now he's stable, sedated. Doctors had waited to see if the bleed on his skull would lead to any further swelling and, thankfully, it did not, which meant he was spared surgery. Even better, by Thursday, the day I visit, they are gradually weaning him off the sedatives and are hopeful that once a chest infection has passed (combated by antibiotics) he'll be able to wake in a matter of days.

'I might be able to beat you on some runs now, Nick,' says Michael Hennessy, Mick's fifteen-year-old son, an amateur boxer.

'No chance,' says Mick.

The promoter now has a dilemma of his own, of course. He's fully aware of his son's ambition to turn professional as a boxer on his eighteenth birthday, but, having seen how much of an impact Nick Blackwell's injury has had on him, Mick feels moved to ask the all-important question (perhaps knowing he'd receive no better shot at getting the answer he wanted): 'Do you *still* want to box, son?'

'Yes, Dad, I do,' says Michael, who, an hour or two after seeing Blackwell leave the ring on a stretcher, was shadowboxing in the hotel lobby of a Holiday Inn. I spotted him. It was then I knew the obsession gripped him, too.

His father's heart sinks. 'Okay,' he says, 'but you have to look after yourself. Hit and not get hit. If you fight any other way, I'm not having it.'

That is their problem. Mine is guilt. I think specifically of Gabriel Ruelas visiting Jimmy Garcia and Rocky Kelly visiting Steve Watt in hospital. I enter their headspace. I didn't damage Nick Blackwell, no, but neither did they deliberately set out to damage – at least not permanently damage – their opponents. Guilt, I realise, doesn't necessarily require intent.

THE RECOVERY

I'm guilty by proxy. I was there. I stirred and promoted the hatred. I wanted a war. I then watched a war and saw Blackwell not as a human being but as something greater. I saw him take punishment and believed it to be entirely natural and acceptable in the context of him carrying out his game plan and slowing down his opponent. I thought, if anyone can take it, *he* can. I made a machine out of him, a disposable hero. Yet now, as I stand by his bedside and think of something to say, Nick Blackwell appears more human than ever. I touch his swollen left hand and leave.

'Get out! You can't stay here! This is not a hotel!' These were just some of the commands shouted at the friends of Nick Blackwell for as long as they claimed the ninth floor of St Mary's adult intensive care unit as their temporary bachelor pad and the designated sitting room as their bedroom. Sleeping in black leather chairs they'd re-labelled 'pods', Jake Jordan, Gareth Heard and Nick's brother, Dan, had ingeniously joined these so-called 'pods' together and used them as beds and were soon wandering the premises half-naked, eating takeaway food, hooking a laptop up to the television to play the latest movies, and washing in the disabled toilets, situated just past reception. How's *that* for dedication? How's *that* for friendship? It was admirable and every bit as humbling as their friend's display of bravery days before. 'I don't give a shit what crap they [hospital staff] come out with,' says Gareth, a trainer and former boxer from Blackwell's old Contender gym. 'We don't want to be away from our friend when he needs us most. If it was jam-packed and everyone was doing the same, I'd understand. But it's not. It's empty.'

Joining the trio in their overly warm bedroom on the day

DOG ROUNDS

I visit are Gary Lockett, Blackwell's trainer, as well as the boxer's father, John, and his younger sister, Hannah. Lockett, a former world middleweight title challenger and one of the best up-and-coming trainers in Britain, has received some unfair criticism, the kind all cornermen in his position receive, but seems to be taking it in his stride. I watch him do impressions, tell anecdotes about Russian gangsters trying to hunt down him and his other fighter, Enzo Maccarinelli, and generally attempt to keep the mood in the room light. An utterly selfless act, none of it is for his own benefit. 'He'll be okay, mate,' he says to me as he detects my concern. 'Seeing him like that shook me up, too. It's horrible, it's haunting, I know. But he looks so much better than he did.'

On the window ledge are some tulips, sent to the boxer by a Turkish family from whom he'd ordered his post-weigh-in meal, and on the table in the middle of the room are numerous empty boxes of food from a local noodle bar, as well as chopsticks, plastic knives, plastic forks and cans of sugar-laden pop. I have, it seems, narrowly missed the feast. Meanwhile, playing on the television is *Escape to the Country*, a BBC show which helps prospective buyers find their pastoral dream home. The Blackwells and friends have grown accustomed to watching daytime television and accept they will be doing so for the foreseeable future. At least until Nick wakes. Today, however, they feel almost at home because featured on *Escape to the Country* are properties in Chippenham, Longleat and Bradford on Avon, none particularly far from Trowbridge. 'That's the Castle Inn Hotel,' says John while sipping from a can of Pepsi.

'Your son will be turning in his bed if he sees you drinking that,' answers Jake, cap on back to front, pointing.

'I know. I don't normally drink it.'

THE RECOVERY

The Hennessys are also present; Mick, the promoter, his wife, Kelly, and two of their three children, Michael and Fran. At one point, to the amusement of those around them, Fran throws punches at the hands of Jake, impressing him with her power and strength, and informs all in the room that she once invited a boy from school to her house for the sole purpose of discovering how tough he was. He had, by all accounts, claimed he was a boxer or wanted to be a boxer and therefore, on that basis, inadvertently declared himself the toughest kid in the playground. Fran, eleven years of age, wanted to prove it. So they gloved up in the Hennessy living room, with Michael as referee, and Fran weathered an early storm, covering up under a fusillade of body and head shots, before crippling the boy with a single hook to the gut.

The retelling of this story has most in fits of laughter, for it is said with great pride and no shortage of enthusiasm, but Mick, the concerned father, is unable to see the funny side of it. 'I tried to keep them away from it,' he says, apologetically. 'Whenever I watched boxing, I'd do it in another room. But one day I came home and there were about six of them sparring in the garden. I said to Michael, "How long have you been doing this?" He said, "Six months." I knew then I had a problem.'

By now, Jake's phone is out and he takes great pleasure in showing sides of Nick, his best mate, affectionately known to him as 'Bing Bong', others might be unfamiliar with. 'You want to see a real side of Nick?' he says. 'He seems like such a tough boxer...' What follows is a short video of Blackwell singing a Britney Spears ballad in a car on his way to Monaco, all the while demonstrating a delicate falsetto. There are many pictures as well. Pictures from Blackwell's fights and from his training camps, pictures of him fat and pictures of him fit. In spite of recent events, it seems there is no hiding from boxing in the sitting room. It hasn't suddenly become an unspoken word. They all discuss it with reverence rather than awkwardness, despite the fact Nick Blackwell, the twenty-five-year-old who links everyone present, will never box again. 'That picture was from the Terry Carruthers fight,' Jake says at one point.

'That Carruthers said he'd never been hit so hard in his life,' adds John, proudly. 'He was bruised to buggery, he was. Nick threw about a thousand punches.'

Jake finishes this brief tour of Nick Blackwell's life, the good, the bad, the embarrassing, with clips of the two of them surfing in Cornwall. Some were taken in Sennen Cove, others in Polzeath, and most feature the boys being dominated by waves far too big for them.

'We met a woman running a crepe and pancake store in Cornwall,' he says. 'She asked Nick, "What do you do for a living?" He said, "I'm a boxer." She didn't understand. She goes, "But how do you make money?" She thought boxing was just a hobby, something he did for fun. The next day we went back there and she said, "I googled you! You *are* a famous boxer! You weren't lying."

'Well, after Nick's fight with Damon Jones on Channel 5, we pulled into a campsite so Nick could go to the toilet and ended up staying there and having a roast dinner. Anyway, as we were at our table, we realised lots of people in the pub were looking at him and talking about him. Turns out many of them had watched his fight on TV. He almost felt famous!'

'They probably only have the five channels in Cornwall,' quips Gareth. 'It just took them a while to catch up.'

'What were the viewing figures like for Saturday, Mick?' Jake asks.

'Very good,' says Mick. 'The best we've had since 2011. Over three million were watching at one point.'

'Brilliant. At the end of the day you're going to want to tune into a fight like that, aren't you? Blood, guts and glory.'

John, the father, returns with an update. He informs all in the room that Nick has been coughing and has taken five breaths on his own.

'He's just kipping,' says Jake. 'We should just put a taser to his nuts. We're supposed to be in Cornwall now surfing.'

Gareth sighs. 'Nick's so inconsiderate.'

Relatively silent in all this is Dan, Nick's brother, exhausted to the point of falling asleep on the floor. He has perhaps been hit hardest by the incident, not only because Nick is his older brother but also because it was only a little over a week ago that he competed in a boxing match of his own. Dan's loss to Dale Coyne at the Victoria Warehouse in Manchester was his sixty-first fight as a professional boxer. It will also be his last.

'I'm going to pack it in,' he tells me. 'I've got a missus and two kids and I can't take the risk. This is a wake-up call for me. If I was single, I might chance it, but I've got a family, I've got a job. It's not worth it.'

Still only twenty-three, Dan's main source of income is the bricklaying trade; the boxing was something he did because he 'enjoyed' it. He had won just seven of his sixty-one fights but was known as one of the very best journeymen on the circuit. Only once had he been stopped (on a cut). He knew how to protect himself better than most.

'When I started out, I wanted to be a contender like Nick,' he says. 'We spar all the time and it's always close. I mean, he has the upper hand, but it's competitive and he has never dropped me or anything. Soon into my career, though, I realised this isn't a sport. The guy I fought on my debut was twelve pounds heavier than me. How is that fair? How is that sport? I lost that one, won my next one, but my record was already looking patchy and it just went downhill from there. Also, you fight some kids and their manager or promoter comes up to you and says, "Hey, he's a bit of a ticket-seller, this lad..." What they mean is, "Go easy on him. Let him win." It's a business, not a sport.'

He tells me he is fond of other sports, like football and fishing, and that he could replace the joy of sparring his brother, Nick, by taking a keener interest in those. They are less dangerous, he says. More fun. 'I have to give up boxing because Nick won't like seeing me carrying on. He'd find that really hard.'

While on the way to see his son in hospital, John Blackwell's phone begins to ring. He looks down at the screen and the number calling is not one he recognises. Momentarily he thinks to ignore it. But then he worries it might be Mick Hennessy, his son's promoter, so decides to go against his gut instinct and answer.

'Hello?' he says.

'What are you doing, Dad?'

John peels the phone from his ear. He stares at it and frowns. He then stares at it again. Harder this time. The voice on the other end sounds like Nick, his son, but how can it be? Nick may have woken from his induced coma on Friday, April Fool's Day no less, but he'd struggled talking over the weekend and was still very much on the road to recovery. Not only that, he'd smashed his mobile phone the week before his fight and was therefore without any form of communication. No, it can't be. No chance. John, a non-believer, accuses Dan, his other son, of pulling a prank on him. He tells him to stop 'pissing about' and to get off the phone.

'Dad, it's me.'

'Okay, then, how did you get a phone?' asks John.

'I'm borrowing one from a nurse.'

Slowly, John starts to believe. 'Oh. Okay. I see. Well, how are you, son?'

'I'm all right, Dad. When are you coming up?'

'In about fifteen minutes.'

'Great. Anyone else coming today?'

'Yeah,' says John. 'Mick, Tyson Fury, a few others.'

'Oh, wicked.'

It is Wednesday, 6 April, and Nick has been awake since Friday. I am told, by John, he has been conversing with friends and posing for pictures in his bed, and he has been walking, and the doctors have even discussed moving him to a hospital closer to home for further rehabilitation. John then beams with pride when describing the moment his son pulled the tube out of his throat, which enabled him to start talking. 'He did it all on his own,' he says. 'The doctors and nurses couldn't believe it.'

Tyson Fury, the reigning heavyweight champion of the world, was the first person Nick had wanted to see, because, in Nick's words, 'He is the only one who will break me out of here.' Nick also informed his friend Jake that he needed to contact Mick Hennessy and ask for a loan, which he'd use to immediately buy himself a safe house, and that he would pay his promoter straight back. For Jake and the others, this confusion, this delirium, was all a bit of fun. They'd use their mate's current state to wind him up. They'd tell him he wasn't in hospital but was, in fact, merely a guest in a

Novotel hotel and that the women who sashayed in and out of his room were waitresses rather than nurses. Blackwell, on the mother of all comedowns, lapped it up. Sometimes he'd pretend he was unconscious, press the emergency button by his bed and watch through squinted eyes as the waitresses rushed into his room, asked his friends what had happened, and then rushed out again. On re-entry, of course, he'd be sat bolt upright, his two thumbs in the air and an almighty grin on his face. The first time it was funny. By the fifth time the waitresses reprimanded him and told him all about the boy who cried wolf.

John has remained in Paddington ever since the incident. He has been staying a five-minute walk around the corner at a nearby hotel. Each morning he visits his son and stays for the duration. 'I haven't been to a car boot sale for three weeks now,' he says, forlornly. 'Before this, I'd hardly missed one in three years.' He points down at his stomach and pinches it. 'And I've been putting on weight. They come in and offer me doughnuts and I think to myself, yeah, why not? But I don't stop at one. I'll have two or three.'

Encouragingly, his son has been getting similar urges. He missed Easter, after all. 'He just wants his roast dinner,' says John. 'He said, "When are we going for roast dinner, Dad?" I said, "What do you want? Beef? Lamb?" He said, "All of it, roasties, the lot." I said, "Okay, son."'

We wait for visiting hours to start. Three to eight o'clock, we are told. I've been here since one. John is used to waiting. He is also by now used to fielding interview requests from newspapers, magazines and television programmes, something which perturbs him no end. '*Good Morning Britain* have asked me to go on their sofa more than once,' he moans. 'It would be with that Jeremy

Kyle. I don't even like the bloke. Nobody wants to hear my Somerset accent anyway.'

At 2:30p.m., John's phone rings. It is another number he fails to recognise.

'Hello?' he says. 'Oh, Nick. Everything all right? I'm in the waiting room. We can't come in until three. Yeah, there's a few people here to see you. We'll be in soon.'

There are three friends waiting to see him and another eight or nine will arrive in the next hour or so. Thanks to my miscalculation, though, I was here first and consequently, just before three o'clock, I am invited by John to walk to the major trauma ward, peel back the door to bed five and see Nick Blackwell as I'd once known him; awake, smiling, two thumbs up. The tubes that once helped him breathe are no more. There are chocolates (a Galaxy bar and a bag of Mini Eggs) and blueberries scattered on his bedside table. He recognises us. He calls us by our names. Questions asked of us are relevant to who we are. He knows all about his friend's dog, for example. He asks about it. He then says that if his own dog, Rosco, was here with him, he'd run in, jump on the bed and probably make him cry. He nearly does just that at the thought alone.

I ask him how he feels. He replies, 'Good, thanks.' He then moves his legs back and forth, bending them at the knee, and says he has been up walking and that his only issue is his left foot, which is currently in a splint and drags a little when on the move. 'It's a bit behind the right,' he says. 'I think where he hit me on the right side of my head, up here,' he points to a spot on his head, 'it messed up my left foot.'

'Can you wiggle your toes, though?'

He can. He does.

More friends pile into the room. There are now five of us in total, including his father, and he greets the newcomers the way he greeted me. He sticks two thumbs up, smiles, addresses them by name and then asks a personal question. How's the football going? How's the missus? That sort of thing.

'What do you remember about the fight?' one of his friends then brazenly asks.

Together, as one, the rest of us hold our breath. I wonder whether questions such as these, questions pertaining to the fight, are coming too soon. A sideways glance is shot the way of Nick's dad. He blinks but that's about it. He allows Nick to talk.

'It was a good fight, a slugfest,' he says. 'He just hit me with a clean shot. I don't remember what shot it was but it must have been a good one.'

Now we all look the way of his father.

'I remember the referee trying to shove veins or straws up my nose and then I tried ripping them out,' Nick continues. 'I was like, "Fuck off!" I didn't want the fight to be stopped. But he obviously hit me with a great shot – in the tenth, wasn't it? – and that was the end of it. It's okay. I'll get my revenge one day.'

He flashes a playful smile which shows he is aware, even at this early stage, that revenge won't come in a boxing ring. He's not delusional. Nor is he foolishly proud. Truly, though, it's hard to stomach the thought that 'Bang Bang' Blackwell believes he has been knocked out by a single blow; for a man renowned for his fitness and durability it is surely a bitter pill to swallow. But nobody thinks to correct him. Frankly, nobody knows quite how to respond. Do we perpetuate this version of events? Is it better if we just nod our heads and agree? Will conflicting opinions only confuse him? Or should one of us speak up and put him straight? Right in the nick of time, John, his father, pulls the plug. He isn't going to have his son thinking he was knocked out by Chris Eubank Jr. Not a chance. 'You weren't knocked out, son,' he says.

'I wasn't?' says Nick.

'You never even went down,' I say. 'You were stopped because of the swelling over your eye.'

Nick, face awash with uncertainty, the truth too much to process, runs his hand over his brow towards the right side of his forehead. 'I thought I could feel a lump here,' he says.

'It was the other side,' says John.

'Oh.'

'Everyone was raving about how tough you were,' I say.

'Really?'

Each of us nod. Never has it felt better to correct someone.

'Apparently people have been raising lots of money for me,' he says.

Confirmation again follows. He is informed of various fundraisers launched by people moved by the incident, one of which raised £12,000, and is then told his Twitter following has soared from 5,000 to 30,000. Jake will even joke that his friend has made more money while in a seven-day coma than he did in his entire seven-year professional boxing career.

'Quite touching, isn't it?' says Nick, rolling his tired head back on a pillow, tears filling his eyes. 'It's like one big family, boxing...'

He, the fighter, has already forgiven it. But only his eventual recovery will allow everyone else implicated, me included, to do the same.

15

LA ADICCIÓN
(THE ADDICTION)

It's a regular Tuesday night in Mexico City. Three masked men floor a fourth man and proceed to stamp all over his head and naked torso, extracting satisfaction not only from the blows but from the smiles on the faces of all who witness this act of violence and soundtrack it with rapturous acclaim. I'm one such bystander, one such voyeur, but there are many others, and rather than scream or cower or, heaven knows, attempt to stop the torrent of abuse, we watch from a safe distance, sat in coloured plastic seats, and find it thoroughly gratifying to see three men manically stomp away on some poor fellow who hasn't the strength nor wherewithal to clamber to his feet or offer any sort of defence. Powerless, his pathetic demise is fully exposed and meant to spark an emotion – call it giddy excitement – in all who have paid money to see it.

Watching a one-sided beatdown is fun.

DOG ROUNDS

That is not a sentence I contemplated writing before visiting Ciudad de México and seeing grown men kick, punch, elbow, head-lock and bite each other in front of a crowd of enthused adults and children, but on this day, this Tuesday evening, it's true. The *act* of violence, or implied violence, as in the case of lucha libre wrestling, is genuinely enjoyable to watch and isn't saddled with the ickiness attached to boxing and other combat sports which also take place in an arena, inside a ring. When seeing it unfold, there is no need for introspection, no need to ask ourselves deep questions regarding the morality of it all. We don't feel guilty. We don't feel ashamed. What a relief.

Seriously, it's absolutely fine to watch grown men *pretend* to beat the shit out of each other. Here, in fact, it's encouraged – by children, by women, by old ladies. They're all having fun. They're being entertained. There are employees of Arena México marching down aisles, interrupting the action and flinging pizza, popcorn, tortillas, crisps, beers, as well as replica masks and capes, the way of anyone naïve enough to make eye contact with them. We crane our necks to see what's happening in the ring, but they take it as a sign of interest and items are duly waved in front of our noses. We shake our heads and feel bad. The kids surrounding us, though, are safer bets. There are scores of them. They purchase the fast food and the masks, then eat the fast food and wear the masks and take pictures on phones of each of the wrestlers making their elaborate entrance to the ring in the middle of the arena. It's in this moment we may as well be at a matinee showing of the latest Pixar film. Kids, popcorn, sugary delights, everywhere. All smiles. The little devils behind the masks and smart phones are seal-clapping with delight and even the wrestlers known as the heels –

the bad guys – carry out their roles with self-deprecation and appear to get a kick out of antagonising the crowd and stoking the hatred. Match over, the heel, the villain, then fist-bumps and high-fives many of the same people who had earlier booed and hissed their every move. It's okay, it's forgiven, it's not real. Forget about it. It's all just pantomime with punches. I quickly begin to love it.

I guess the clue lies in the *mascara* (the mask). It's the concealer, the cover-up, and behind it normal Mexicans, and some international wrestlers, are able to play roles, act up, and mimic with gusto actions commonly associated with assault charges elsewhere in the world. Because of these masks, we *all* feel safe, as the spectacle takes on a kind of otherworldliness which means we can only laugh; masks come in all colours, shapes and sizes, some shinier and snazzier than others, and help create the fantasy to which we surrender our preconceptions. The wrestlers donning them are similarly ludicrous. Nitro's is red and black, accompanied by a suit of armour and a black-and-white native American poncho and red Lycra pants, while Magnus goes for an army camouflage and gold mask with a gold cape, removed on the runway, and Oro Jr chooses black and gold for his mask and a matching leather cape, which is left open for all to assess his abdominal muscles. They all look utterly comical. But they don't care. Even the ones spared the mask are just as amusing to the eye. Canelo Casas flings his long black hair around like a propeller, all the while snugly stuffed into a red leather waistcoat, and Leono's bleach-blond hair, circular shades and sleeveless black shirt and long white scarf bring to mind a confused lovechild of Hogan, Flair and Savage. Then there's Metálico, my personal favourite. He has come dressed as a cowboy, complete with a green checked shirt and hat, and saunters down the runway serenading the crowd and dancing with four scantily clad ring-card girls. Though I warm to him, Metálico is unquestionably a heel. He is designed to be booed, he wants to be booed and he does all he can to ensure he is booed, which is to say he berates the referee, riles the crowd, complains of foul moves, cries injury and generally plays the old, whinging killjoy, as if it's not much of a stretch. The crowd, of course, harangue him for it. They boo and hiss and stamp their feet in accordance to the rules. They want their wrestlers to wrestle. They want their fighters to fight. There is no room in their hearts for those who bleat and do everything in their power *not* to fight. Metálico, I'm afraid to say, is the anti-warrior. He's here to enrage rather than engage; midway through the action, when figuratively and occasionally literally getting his behind kicked, he moans of a leg cramp and skedaddles, much to the audience's dismay.

There are, in truth, only a thousand or so Mexicans in the venue – a building that holds 16,000 – but more will arrive closer to the main event and they too will possess the same looks of wonder and admiration, for the acrobatics and the choreography, and then release the stresses of the week on the men in masks created and willing to soak up their pseudo-hatred. They'll spit rage their way, wag their fingers at them, pray the heels get their comeuppance, and then belly laugh about it afterwards. It all feels, to me, like violence done right. Violence for all the family. Nobody's getting hurt out here. Not *really* hurt. These guys are simply playing dress-up. So sit back, relax and enjoy the show. Here's a slice of Domino's pizza. Fifty pesos.

Now for the unmasking, if you will. On 20 March 2015, Perro Aguayo Jr played dress-up with Rey Mysterio Jr, Manik and Xtreme Tiger in Tijuana, Baja California, Mexico, only to pay the ultimate price. A Mysterio head-scissor takedown propelled him out of the ring and then, on his return, he was dropkicked by Mysterio in the shoulder, a shot used to set up Mysterio's signature 619 move. The kick left him prostrate on the middle rope, head and arms dangling in front of him, perfectly positioned for the 619, yet Aguayo was seemingly unconscious; this, it goes without saying, was obviously not part of the plan. Manik, one of the other wrestlers, fell on to the middle rope beside Aguayo and fleetingly glanced his way. Was he acting? The match went on.

Mysterio, to the delight of the Mexican fans, performed his 619, grabbing the middle ropes with his hands and then swinging out of the ring and back in again with both legs, but missed Aguayo and Manik on re-entry. Manik checked on Aguayo, sensing something wasn't right, and watched as he slumped to the bottom rope, his head banging the canvas en route. Was he *still* acting? The match went on.

Manik left Aguayo's side and was promptly kicked by Xtreme Tiger, as per the script, and Xtreme Tiger then clapped his hands and roused the audience. He leaped outside the ring and continued his scrap with Manik in full view of the crowd. Mysterio, at this point, held Aguayo's T-shirt from behind and checked on him. It didn't look like acting any more. He alerted the referee. The match went on.

Moments later, Mysterio performed another 619, this time connecting on Manik, who was positioned next to a prone and now completely horizontal Aguayo, and swiftly set up the finishing move. The match went on until it was finished by Mysterio pinning Manik.

By now many around ringside knew something was wrong. Konnan, a fellow wrestler, attempted to revive Aguayo by shaking him back to consciousness and others followed suit once the match concluded. At the time, ringside physicians were backstage treating other wrestlers who had been injured that night, one of whom had a spine injury, and this meant Aguayo lacked immediate and proper medical attention. It also meant he left the ring on a bit of plywood as opposed to a stretcher.

Aguayo, thirty-five, was eventually taken to the local Del Prado hospital and pronounced dead at around one o'clock on the morning of 21 March 2015. Cause of death was initially deemed a cervical spine trauma, reportedly a result of Mysterio's dropkick catapulting him forward to the ring ropes and the ropes then snapping his neck, something that brought to mind Michael Watson and Chris Eubank's uppercut. But, in time, the actual cause of Aguayo's death was pinpointed as a cardiac arrest resulting from a cervical stroke. He had three fractured vertebrae, at C1, C2 and C3, and the coroner revealed the fractures occurred at two different moments of impact. He said Aguayo died almost instantly.

During the fall-out, the attorney general for Baja California announced they would conduct an investigation into the death to determine whether or not criminal charges should be filed. Mysterio, meanwhile, received threats and was called a 'killer', yet, on 23 March, the day Aguayo was buried in Guadalajara, he served as one of the pallbearers, before later declaring his intention to continue wrestling. It was, he said, what Aguayo, his friend, would have wanted.

Video clips of this lucha libre death can be found on YouTube and have been watched by well over four million people. It's a glimpse of shocking tragedy, so there will naturally be interest, but it's also intriguing to many by virtue of the fact it occurred within a world of spandex make-believe. In a business where the name of the game is to pretend, to not *really* hurt or get hurt, how did some poor man lose his life? Lucha libre is meant to be fun, a child-friendly alternative to fight sports, and its art lies in the ability of the luchadores to not hurt their opponent but merely appear as if they are doing so. Yet even in lucha libre, a spectacle governed not only by a referee and rules but by its participants' trained ability to avoid proper violence, death still occurs. How's that pizza?

Back in Mexico City, my wife, Louisa, and I watch the first few matches and then leave just before the main event title fight between Máximo Sexy and Rey Escorpión. My wife uses any excuse she can muster to escape the incessant, droning shouts of 'Tortas! Papas! Cerveza!' and I'm also keen to flee. In agreement, we squeeze past overweight, sugar-fuelled, masked Mexican kids and reach the exit aisle just after nine o'clock. Soon enough we're outside in the pouring rain being flogged tickets (for the next lucha libre event on Friday), T-shirts and tacos.

I wish I could say we decided to depart early in some kind of (admittedly pointless) tribute to Perro Aguayo Jr. That we got on our high horses and, giddy up, rode out of there, informing anyone who questioned our premature exit that a man once died doing the very thing they dared to enjoy on a Tuesday evening. We'd remind them he died in the ring and that wrestlers continued to wrestle and that people, *you people*, continued to cheer and clap and mock and eat popcorn and drink Corona. 619? How about 911?

But, in truth, nothing of the sort entered our minds. Instead, after two-and-a-half hours inside Arena México, boredom had set in. We'd seen enough. We'd covered all types of masks, all types of entrances, all types of characters, all types of moves, and simply had our fill of the process, the theatrics, the leather, the Lycra. And, honestly, though it's written with no pride whatsoever, I genuinely wanted to see someone throw and connect with a punch. A solid, hurtful, *real* punch. I wanted it all to mean something.

Inside the Azteca Boxing Club in La Paz, Mexico, punches are the order of the day as fighters spar in a miniature thirteen-by-thirteen-foot ring and get intimate through violence. There is little room to breathe, much less move. Raúl Hirales, the gym's owner and super-bantamweight-cum-featherweight contender, works out with a sparring partner and fists flow freely. Hands move in a manner feet cannot, and the two boxers stay connected and work angles and space via head and upper-body movement rather than shifting position, for this is the Mexican way. Thirteen-foot rings encourage it, machismo prolongs it, and the sweltering heat inside the converted garage – located next to a sushi shack across the road from a printing shop – intensifies it.

Boxers dip out of the gym and stand on the roadside, gloves still on hands, gum shield still in mouth, just to suck in some air. One of them, thirty-two-year-old Hirales, weighing 135 pounds before the session, seeks refuge in the street and says he has already, in the past half an hour, lost five pounds on his journey down to the featherweight limit of 126. It's easy to believe him. The heat suffocates. It weakens. There are six old fans on the ceiling above our heads but only five work. Testament to the heat, Hirales' arms are sinewy, every one of the veins in his forearms prominent, and his face, golden and chiselled, cheekbones so sharp they're surely a hazard in a clinch, moves my wife, a superb judge of character, to label him the most handsome boxer she has ever seen.

LA ADICCIÓN (THE ADDICTION)

There are three other fighters in the gym, one of whom is former IBF world minimumweight champion Raúl García, but none grab the attention like the diminutive bronze figure in luminous green hand-wraps and a blue Puma T-shirt. He spars two of the others, and they rattle through six rounds. They are the first rounds I have seen Raúl complete since I sat ringside and watched him box in Nottingham, England, in 2012. He faced Ireland's Carl Frampton that May night and lost a unanimous decision after twelve rounds. Raúl was undefeated beforehand, without a setback in seventeen bouts, but found the travelling and the step up in class too much. 'Frampton was very strong,' he tells me. 'In previous fights, I watched him come forward and fight aggressively, on the front foot, pushing forward, but, when I fought him, he went on the back foot. That surprised me.'

Raúl's father, overseeing today's sparring session, pulls up a picture of his son and Frampton on his mobile phone. The image depicts the two boxers in a warm post-fight embrace. It also shows Frampton with various swellings and scuff marks on his face, perhaps a sign the fight was tougher than the judges' scorecards reflected, and thus a moral victory of sorts, especially given Frampton's subsequent rise to prominence as a world champion. Furthermore, there's a hint, in the picture, a flashback to carefree, idealistic times, of a very different Raúl Hirales; four years younger, ambitious, gunning for a world title, even in defeat he had a bright future ahead of him, as self-belief and the naivety of youth continued to act as fuel.

But then, on 19 October 2013, he boxed a fellow Mexican and former amateur teammate, Francisco Leal, and the Raúl Hirales in the picture on his father's phone – battered, beaten but beaming and still full of hope – was soon to fade.

DOG ROUNDS

The Leal fight, which took place in Cabo San Lucas, Mexico, ended in the eighth round when Leal was sent to the canvas by a series of right hands and was unable to stand without the assistance of the ropes. Unresponsive, he slumped to the canvas thereafter, as efforts to keep him upright were futile, before slipping in and out of consciousness while propped up against the corner post.

Hirales' celebration, which was instinctively jubilant, simmered and was replaced by a haunted stare into the middle distance. He winced upon seeing Leal horizontal and placed on a stretcher. It was fast turning ugly and he knew it; everybody aware of the signs knew it. Frankie Leal was going to pass away just three days before his twenty-seventh birthday and there was nothing anybody could do to prevent it.

Hirales, an active fighter, now lives and breathes the kind of career many of the men in this book have detailed from a comfier position of retrospection. He has lost his last three fights, all via decision, all because he didn't turn up the heat and do enough, and the dream of one day winning a world title now appears entirely unrealistic even if he must convince himself setbacks lead to comebacks and that it's all a learning curve and that one day the trials and tribulations will bear fruit and so on and so forth (insert additional fighter clichés). Were I to encounter Raúl Hirales in ten years' time, when his fragile hands are no longer wrapped and he's busy making money elsewhere, he may well view the Leal tragedy and his subsequent career trajectory in very different terms. Truer terms. He might accept he was never the same fighter from that day forth. He might even concede the tragedy ruined him. But for as long as he remains active and trying – his next fight is just six weeks away – he has no choice but to combine a little honesty with a lot of delusion. It's how he gets through the day. It's how he's still able to punch men in the face.

So what of the sparring? Well, for starters, a thirteen-by-thirteen-foot ring, no place for pacifists, is about as unforgiving as any arena in which two men can swap blows. Therefore, even if a boxer is at all reticent, it's mightily hard for them to escape. Raúl, for the record, certainly doesn't hide. He throws both hands to head and body and showcases every conceivable shot in the book. He comes forward aggressively. He upholds the Mexican tradition. Yet, what *is* noticeable is how he reduces the snap in his punches, almost placing them rather than powering through and finishing them, and how he seems to just be playing in there, putting on a demonstration, going through the motions, as opposed to asserting himself and claiming the upper hand. Maybe this is simply because he's more experienced than the boxers with whom he spars. Or maybe it's because he views sparring only as practice. Maybe it's a bit of both. Maybe it's something else entirely. What's clear, though, is that he is undoubtedly tuned down and nowhere near as sprightly as I remember him being in Nottingham four years ago.

He calls it experience. He *has* to call it that. 'I'm improving with age because I'm gaining experience,' Raúl says after sparring, as he prepares to slug one of the seven black heavy bags located towards the rear of the gym. 'The next fight is very important to me because I haven't fought in over a year and I'm facing a good prospect. I need a win. The layoff has been very frustrating. It wasn't my fault. Boxing is my way of life. It's how I earn money and support my family. Without boxing, I can't provide.'

DOG ROUNDS

Raúl has been boxing since the age of eight, influenced by his father, a long-time boxing coach, but concedes his wife is keen to see him quit. She doesn't like watching him fight and has only personally attended one of his bouts. Usually she waits at home for a text message to reveal the result. Raúl, though, warns it will be this way for a little while yet. 'I will probably fight for three or four more years, hopefully,' he says. 'I'm improving with experience and trying to adapt and do different types of training. I still have the ambition of one day winning a title.'

There's that word again. *Experience*. It's an alternative, softer way of saying time is passing. Raúl knows this, as all boxers know this. Stick with 'experience' and hope resumes. It's all about self-preservation, you see. Buzzwords are their *mascara*. Not that Hirales is a lost cause, nor living in a permanent state of fantasy or denial. If that were the case, he wouldn't have images of Frankie Leal lining the walls of his gymnasium and he wouldn't possess a framed fight report from the bout in question. No, Hirales, in keeping with his fighting style, refuses to run. He won't hide from the thing that has changed him and soured something he has done since childhood. Mentally, at least, he's trying to deal with it. Signs are everywhere. Scan the gym walls and you'll find, painted in black ink and supported by an image of two Reyes boxing gloves, the following rallying cry:

Colgar los guantes
seria lo más facil
lo más sencillo
peros jamás
lo más correcto
vamos

LA ADICCIÓN (THE ADDICTION)

No puedes rendirte ahora
Lucha una vez más

The message, when translated into English, says that hanging up the gloves would be the easiest option but that it's never the right thing to do and that he must fight again. Raúl expands on this when he wraps up the day's training session and invites me to taste the sea food at Chocolatas El Empanada, located not far from the Malecón. I settle for the shrimp ceviche, while he goes for a plastic cup containing clams in tomato juice. Over raw fish I bring up Frankie Leal, a subject he rarely discusses with anyone but his psychologist.

'I went to therapy after the Frankie Leal fight,' he says. 'It was something I did as an amateur when the national team provided psychologists for the boxers. I go to see them now and again when I feel like I need to. I go quite a lot if I've got a fight coming up; when I feel there's a problem, I'll go. We talk about lots of different things, lots of personal things, but the Leal fight is always one of the main things we discuss.'

'Whose decision was it to seek out therapy?' I ask.

'It was my decision and also my family's. I go to a therapist in La Paz and also converse with the therapist I had in the amateurs on Facebook. It's now part of my fight preparation.'

'How much did the death of Frankie Leal affect you?'

'It affected me a lot. Outside the ring we were really good friends, Frankie and I, but we both knew what happens when we get inside the ring. Then it's time to fight. It's completely different. We can make that switch from friends to opponents. That's what we did. That made it so much harder.'

'What do you remember about the fight?'

'It was quite an equal fight and the end was something

quite sudden. I remember it was really hot. I don't think the heat helped either of us that night.'

'Were you the same fighter after that?' I ask, stifling my own thoughts on the matter.

'No,' he says. 'I didn't put so much pressure on my next opponent [Fernando Vargas]. When I was hitting him, I was kind of holding back a little. I was worried and feared it might happen to my opponent again and that it might happen to me, too. It was a reminder of how dangerous boxing can be. I hadn't thought about its dangers before.'

Therapy, he would go on to say, has changed his mindset somewhat, helped him recover, and is the reason he is back to something like his best, despite three defeats on the spin. Without therapy, he'd be left with no choice but to concede defeat and retire, an inconceivable thought with a wife and three children to support.

'Would you want your children to box?' I ask him.

Raúl shakes his head, then smiles.

'Why not?'

'It's not the danger,' he says, quick to end my prodding of that particular spot. 'There's a lot of sacrifice. It's a tough sport. You've got to leave your family and dedicate your life to it.'

'Do you enjoy boxing?'

He nods.

'What aspects?'

'The running and the diet, not so much. Everything else is okay, though. I couldn't contemplate a life without boxing. Even though I thought about leaving, I couldn't bring myself to do it. This is what I like to do. I'm addicted to it.'

'Addictions can kill,' I say. 'Do you fear the same thing happening to you?'

LA ADICCIÓN (THE ADDICTION)

'I never thought about it before,' he says, 'but, curiously, after my fight with Frankie Leal, it started to happen elsewhere in other fights. It happened to Óscar González. There were others, too. It makes you realise it can happen to anyone.'

Óscar González was another Hirales opponent – he faced him in December 2012 – who passed away as a result of injuries suffered in a boxing ring. Jesús 'Zurdo' Galicia stopped González in round ten of a fight in Mexico City in February 2014 and the fighter known as 'Fantasma', or 'The Ghost', died two days later. Understandably, for Hirales, a man who traded hurtful blows with both Leal *and* González, it was an eerie turn of events, something that would regrettably link him to a death in the ring not once but twice. But what made it worse, particularly in the case of Frankie Leal, is that Raúl Hirales should probably never have shared the ring with him in the first place. After all, Leal, nicknamed 'Little Soldier' and boasting a record of twenty wins, eight losses and three draws, had been badly knocked out in the tenth round by Russia's Evgeny Gradovich in March 2012, a defeat which saw him exit the ring on a stretcher and end up in hospital only to return to action less than a year later. Not long after that he was dead.

If only he had replicated the thought process of American super-bantamweight Al Seeger, who begrudgingly retired in 2009 following a fractured skull in his final fight. Look up the injury and you'll see why. You'll also discover a stomach-churning image of a man's bruised and bloodied forehead out of which an upside-down triangle, almost a miniature pizza slice, seems to have been carved, a medical stencil pulling the outlying skin down to reveal cogs and mesh, like the inside of a clock, where the skin should be, as ran by *South Magazine* alongside an article titled 'The Comeback of Al Seeger'. It's a jarring picture, enough to make even a cannibal queasy. It's also a shocking indictment of how dangerous and gruesome the sport of boxing can be, as well as a reminder, if ever one was needed, of why Al Seeger had no choice but to hang up the gloves. Spoiler alert: there would be no comeback, despite what the headline writers inferred. And how could there be? Seeger's forehead, in the area where the sinus is located, had been pushed backwards and the plastic surgeon, Dr Bill Dascombe, said the damage was comparable to the type of injury encountered by someone who falls off a horse or is cast from an all-terrain vehicle. There was also blood found on Seeger's brain. Forget boxing, he was lucky just to be alive.

Ask him how it happened and he'll go one better than that. He'll tell you *when*. It happened, he says, the moment Victor Fonseca, his final opponent, head-butted him in round two of an NABF super-bantamweight title fight on 23 October 2009. He heard the crack, he felt the pain. Watching the fight back, he even noticed the subsequent indentation on his forehead, the result of his sinus cavity being collapsed; once the cavity was smashed, every follow-up blow contained a far greater danger and felt like an anvil being struck against his forehead. But Seeger still carried on in the fight. He made it through rounds three, four, five, six, seven and eight, winning many of them, before being stopped in the ninth. He was ahead on two of the three scorecards at the time and remains adamant head-butts rather than punches did most of the dirty work.

'I've been head-butted before but never felt the way I did that night,' he recalls. 'It was a different sort of pain, a different sort of sensation, and we cracked heads a couple of times after that and it made it worse. Honestly, it was like a light went off in the end. It wasn't any particular punch that finished me. The damage was done.'

During his ambulance ride to Laredo hospital, Seeger would lean his head back and feel it fill up with blood. He'd then lean forward and the blood would pour from his nose. Something was wrong, that much was obvious, but the idea that he might be dealing with a blood spot on his brain, caused by the reckless head-butts of his opponent, was simply too much to bear. Jimmy Chumley, his long-time trainer, sat beside Al and shook his head. 'Man, this is it,' he said. 'I'm not doing this shit any more.'

Out of the intensive care unit, and resting in a regular hospital room, Seeger considered his own fighting future while waiting for a small metal plate to be implanted above his nose and between his eyebrows. It was presumably at this point, before being flown by helicopter to San Antonio University Hospital for surgery, he remembered he'd made a paltry $7,000 for fighting Fonseca. 'That surgery was the worst pain I'd ever had in my life,' Al says. 'Like a nail going into my head, man.'

The doctors, upon viewing the scans, reiterated to Al how lucky he was to still be alive, but the fighter initially wanted more than to just be alive. He was angry and frustrated, a wronged man. He needed to exact revenge on Fonseca, punish him for his indiscretions, and get back in the hunt for titles. He had so much more he wanted to do. He was only twenty-nine.

And so, in spite of the fractured skull, broken sinus cavity, broken frontal bone and subdural haematoma behind his ear, and in spite of the impassioned pleas from Jimmy Chumley for him to retire, Seeger was insistent he would fight again. He went back to the gym, he hit the bag, he hit pads, he even began to spar, just like the old days, moving around with the best fighters available. But then came the nose bleeds caused by friction from the screws on the plate grinding against the inside of his head. They stemmed from innocuous moments – taps on the face, half-hearted shots to the head – and, once his nose started streaming, it was near impossible to stop. 'I could spar big guys in the gym and not feel a thing, and then I could get in there with a twelve-year-old girl and she'd hit me on the sweet spot and that nose would bleed everywhere.' This happened time and time again. It was no freak occurrence. Al had become fragile overnight. He was now vulnerable in the ring.

If in any doubt, a doctor from the New York Athletic Commission phoned him and offered his thoughts on the matter. He advised Al to retire on account of the haematoma he had suffered in the fight with Fonseca and then explained to him that if an athlete is unfortunate enough to suffer one the likelihood of them developing another goes up considerably. In other words, Seeger was now considered damaged goods. 'When Benjamin Flores died, my brother said it might be a sign,' Al says. 'But I didn't think like that. I couldn't afford to. This was a wake-up call for me, though. It was almost like I was forced out of boxing – for a reason. Somebody didn't want me in the sport any more.'

Here's the thing. Al Seeger knew the dangers of boxing better than most because Benjamin Flores, a twenty-four-year-old Mexican, died two days after Seeger had stopped him in an NABF super-bantamweight title fight on 30 April 2009. The incident crushed Al. It took something away from him. It led to Ray 'Boom Boom' Mancini picking up the phone to advise him. And it wasn't just that, either. Al Seeger also knew the dangers of boxing better than most because he'd been warned of them ever since setting foot inside Jarrell's Gym in Savannah as a young boy.

'Are y'all ready for tomorrow night?' his coach, Mike Jarrell, would enquire as a swarm of amateur boxers gathered in his office before a night of fights the next day. 'Yeah!' they replied as one, fist-pumping the air, bouncing on their toes, getting in the zone. 'Are you ready to die in there?' he would ask next. This time the response was understandably less vociferous. Some nervously looked the other way. Others bowed their heads. Most stayed silent. Little Al Seeger was one of the few, however, who responded with just as much zeal and certainty as he did when answering the first question. He was damn sure of it.

'I never hesitated,' he says many years later. 'I was the first one to shout "yeah" back and I told myself, "If I've got to die, I've got to die." I was willing to die in the ring. There's no better way to die than to die doing something you love. So, I accepted my fate. I knew there was a chance I could be badly injured or worse each time I stepped into the ring and I was fine with that. It was a risk I was willing to take. Death was the last thing I'd want to happen, to either me or my opponent, but it wasn't anything that was going to make me think twice about boxing.'

Seeger boxed thirty-three times as a professional and before nearly every one of those fights he'd create a journal, a fight log, in which he'd include details of training, his diet, his thoughts on his opponent, game plans and so on. It was a running commentary of his career and would let him know what he was doing right or wrong, for his own peace of mind. There was a meticulousness to it, too. The game plans wouldn't just be general overviews, they'd be round-by-round breakdowns of what he intended to do on fight night, and each time he finished a journal entry he'd add a note at the bottom which informed whoever found the journal that Al Seeger had died doing what he loved to do and that he would see them again soon. He begged them not to be mad. He reminded them he knew what he was signing up to, that it was meant to be this way. You know, just in case.

Seeger was never afraid of death. He still isn't. Even now his favourite place to chill is the Catholic Cemetery in Savannah, located just off the main street by Shuman Elementary School. It's where he hangs out with his three children, Austin, Atticus and Aloys, and it's where he used to do his roadwork before fights. The relationship between Seeger and death has long been tight. He's learnt to accept it, embrace it.

The same cannot be said of Flores and Leal and González, three young Mexican boxers who died within the space of five years, three young Mexican boxers who were ultimately oblivious to it.

'Why is boxing in Mexico so popular?' I ask Raúl Hirales in La Paz.

He says it's because Mexicans are *guerreros*, or warriors, and then repeats his answer from earlier. 'We're addicted to fighting.'

Before leaving Baja California Sur, I take a trip to Auditorio Municipal in Cabo San Lucas, the outdoor venue in which Hirales defeated Leal in 2013, and discover a serene basketball court covered by a concrete ceiling, allowing light in from all sides, and five Mexican kids practising lay-ups and destined-to-fail dunks and alley-oops. Further down the court are a couple of hefty men going through yoga routines on mats, while outside the venue is a baseball field and a football pitch, both with floodlights, and a sublime view of the local hills and sea.

The sport of boxing, at this moment in time, couldn't be less relevant. There are no signs of it. There is no room for it, no place for it. And yet, unbeknown to the boys enthusiastically bouncing an orange ball up and down, ostensibly playing a game, Frankie Leal, a prizefighter, once fought for his life at half-court. 'I have no problem returning,' Raúl says. 'I have been back before and it doesn't affect me. There's a hospital on the highway, though, quite close by, and that affects me. It was where I visited Frankie.'

'What was that like?' I ask.

'It was horrible seeing him in that condition. I wanted him to talk, say something. I told him his son was waiting for him and that he should keep fighting.'

As I watch smiling kids try with all their might to ambitiously sink three-pointers from beyond the arc, I ponder how different life would have been for Frankie Leal had he frequented the Auditorio Municipal as a young point-guard or even as a pitcher or centre-forward. How simpler life could have been. How longer his life could have been. I then have similar thoughts in Mexico City when seeing two young boys at a bus stop late at night wearing boxing hand wraps. On their way to a life of pain, they mess around and throw punches at one another's midsection and the scene acts as a reminder of Raúl's words; the *guerreros*, the addiction. Soon more kids will appear, only these kids wear ripped vests and have dirt around their eyes, and they walk on the road, slaloming between cars, and they sell sweets and cigars and perform tricks with footballs and juggling balls in the hope of scoring a few pesos in the time it takes for the traffic lights to flick from red to green.

It's then you realise, maybe Frankie Leal died doing the thing he loved.

16

THE ANOMALY

They nearly all, to a man, have rough first fights back. That much is a given. The more pertinent question, I suppose, and the one asked of me more than any other is the following: which boxer, having killed an opponent in the ring, has then been able to go on and make a success of themselves in the sport? To that question, I respond with one name: Barry McGuigan. It's an answer that usually generates a look of disbelief on the face of whoever initiated the conversation. 'Barry McGuigan killed someone in the ring?' they say, incredulous. 'I never knew that.'

It happened on 14 June 1982 at The Grosvenor House Hotel, inside the so-called Great Room. McGuigan was just twenty-one years of age at the time. It was only his twelfth professional fight. The opponent was a Nigerian called Asymin Mustapha who fought under the catchier moniker of Young Ali. His bout with McGuigan plainly marked a considerable step-up in class for the twenty-one-year-old featherweight. It would also, however, guarantee a pay cheque, as good a reason as any to give and take punches.

For Belfast's McGuigan, the 1978 Commonwealth Games gold medallist, Ali was just another faceless opponent, a tune-up ahead of a shot at the British featherweight title, another name on what he hoped would be a long and illustrious list. 'He looked tough. That was my first impression,' McGuigan tells me at The Butcher & Grill in Battersea. 'Tall with plenty to hit, but tough. I remember hitting him with everything and couldn't budge him. I shook him a few times but he had very good powers of recovery. I was winning the rounds, but not by much. I wasn't beating him from pillar to post or anything like that.'

Young Ali sat down in his corner at the conclusion of round five and motioned to his cornerman that his jaw felt strange. 'I can't feel it,' he said. 'It feels like it's floating around.' The cornerman, in the heat of battle, did what many would and brushed off the concern with a frown and a shake of the head. He encouraged his flagging fighter and sent him out for round six.

Thirty-three years later, McGuigan demonstrates the trajectory of the final punch, the right hand, as though it has stayed with him all this time. 'I hit him,' he says, smashing his right fist into the palm of his left hand, 'right on the nose, and his eyes just rolled back.' He shakes his head. 'I remember looking at his eyes rolling back so clearly. It was a haunting moment. I knew he wasn't going to get up from that. It wasn't a normal knockdown. He was down on his face. The way he reacted wasn't good. But then he didn't get up at all. He never regained consciousness after that punch.'

THE ANOMALY

Amid the ensuing panic, a number of people retrieved a spread, a cloth, from one of the tables outside the ring and used it to produce a makeshift stretcher. They folded the spread and pulled it tight, real tight, and would try to keep it as flat and as straight as they could in order to remove Ali's body from the ring. But worse than a makeshift stretcher pulled tight from a table cloth, in 1982 there was no established protocol for when a boxer was injured. It was all improvisation, an attempt to make the best out of a bad situation. Consequently, Young Ali had to wait – yes, *wait* – for an ambulance to arrive before then being taken to the nearest hospital, rather than a neurosurgical hospital, which, nowadays, would be informed in advance that a professional boxing event was taking place and be on red alert for potential head injuries. There were no such pre-emptive measures back in 1982. Young Ali may as well have just been a civilian that night, a civilian who'd taken a heavy punch and suffered a fall outside a nightclub, for there was no stretcher, no paramedics, no ambulance, no neurosurgical hospital and no anaesthetist at ringside, something else which is mandatory today. He was taken to one hospital, registered with the hospital, then sent to another. With each move, he lost valuable minutes.

They eventually scanned Young Ali's head to find the bleeding, shaved his head, cut into the skull, removed the skull cap and then attempted to fuse the bleed. After that, they left the skull open, so the brain could swell and then come back down again, before putting the skull cap back on.

Roughly a month later, Ali was sent home in a comatose state to Nigeria and kept alive on a respirator. In that time, McGuigan discovered a bit more about his story. He found out his wife was pregnant and that he'd made the trip to

London to source money for her. McGuigan's wife, Sandra, was also pregnant, a coincidence that not only tightened Barry's bond to Ali but also broke his heart, for there was now a very real chance only one of the two young boxers would live to see their newborn child.

'It was in a hotel, it was a low-key occasion and there was no television coverage, so they tried sweeping it under the carpet a bit,' McGuigan says. 'But for me, as a sensitive kid, it was never going to go away. I thought, fuck, what am I involved in here? What sort of game is this? Jesus Chris, this kid died in the ring with me. Do I really want to be involved in this? I never wanted to kill anybody. I never wanted to hurt someone like that. I genuinely didn't think I was cut out for the sport. But what else could I do? I thought, well, hold on, Barry, you're not qualified for anything else. You're twenty-one years old. You've got a promising career ahead of you. You've invested all of your eggs in one basket. That's all you've got. Also, my wife was heavily pregnant, as was his...' McGuigan stops to compose himself. Tears accumulate in his eyes and he uses a hand to wipe them away. 'Sandra was doing six days a week in the hairdressing salon because I was still a prospect and earning very little money. What could I do? Did I want to go and learn to become a hairdresser? Did I want to become a PE teacher? Did I want to go back to school? The more I thought about it, the more I knew I had to box. Listen, I know it was a tragic accident – I *know* it was – and I know it could so easily have been me, but I had put far too much into boxing to turn my back on it. I said, right, I'm going to go full-blast and give it everything. And if I ever get to fight for a world title, he'll be the first one on my mind.'

Before any heartfelt world title dedications, McGuigan first had to get back in the ring and punch another man to the head and body, just as he'd once done to Young Ali, and in doing so revisit feelings of ferocity and spite he now considered long-lost friends. His comeback opponent, four months later, was 'Jumping' Jimmy Duncan, a novice featherweight from Liverpool, who McGuigan battled at the Ulster Hall and hurt, badly, in the third round. Woozy, out on his feet, and lacking the energy to mount any kind of retaliation, Duncan was ready to be taken. He was primed to be finished. The crowd, on their feet, willed McGuigan to do just that. Finish him.

But McGuigan, for obvious reasons, wasn't in a finishing mood that night. To the crowd's dismay, he hesitated. He stopped altogether. Then, while in the process of dilly-dallying, he copped a left hook and his head started spinning. 'I suddenly thought, Jesus!' he says. 'I took ten seconds to gather my thoughts and got out of there.'

Once back in the corner, McGuigan faced up to his trainer, Eddie Shaw, and prepared himself for the barrage.

'What the hell was all that about?' Shaw asked.

'It's nothing, Eddie,' replied McGuigan.

'Well, don't fucking do it again, okay?'

The fighter nodded. His head was straight. A round later, the fight was over. McGuigan stopped Duncan. 'I never had that moment's hesitation before,' he says. 'I didn't like it. I didn't feel good in there. But it quickly disappeared.'

The Duncan left hook, a cautionary warning, was all that was required. His next fight, his fourteenth, was just a month later, again at Ulster Hall, against the undefeated Paul Huggins. It was the British title eliminator he'd been building towards. McGuigan, back to something like his best, won it in round five.

Soon after, however, the news they'd all been dreading finally emerged from Nigeria. On 13 December 1982, Young

DOG ROUNDS

Ali, also known as Asymin Mustapha, passed away, having been in a coma for six months.

'It was horrible,' McGuigan says. 'How could I *not* feel guilty? Here I was, a popular young boxer, someone who people admired, and I'd killed someone. I think about the kid all the time. I think about how things could have been different. And I still pray for him as often as I can.'

'But do you *still* feel guilty or responsible for what happened?' I ask McGuigan.

He frowns, glances at the table, then meets my stare. 'I always felt I was more compassionate than most fighters. But I had a killer instinct and it was that killer instinct which ended many of my fights within the distance. Young Ali was no different, and that's what distressed me. I took him out, without hesitation, and finished him when I sensed he was hurt. That's something I'll struggle with for the rest of my life.'

McGuigan, fifty-four, now calls himself one of the lucky ones. He does so for a number of reasons. Lucky because he retired at twenty-eight with his faculties intact. Lucky because he has been able to flourish in retirement – promote fighters, manage fighters, commentate on fights – and make a second living from the sport. Lucky most of all, though, because he is defined not by the death of Young Ali but by a win over Panamanian great Eusebio Pedroza at Queens Park Rangers' Loftus Road Stadium on 8 June 1985. You know it. You've heard about it. It was the night McGuigan's father, Pat, sang 'Danny Boy' as part of the pre-fight introductions. It was the night a raucous live crowd of twenty-six thousand, twelve thousand of which were Irish, as well as nineteen million people watching at home on terrestrial television, saluted a new star of British boxing. It was the night McGuigan, then

238

twenty-four, out-hustled a brilliant champion, someone with nineteen consecutive title defences to his name, someone unbeaten in nine years, for fifteen rounds. It was the night McGuigan became WBA world featherweight champion. It is the night he is asked about more than any other.

Three years on from Young Ali, and sixteen fights later, 8 June 1985 was the night McGuigan paid tribute via a memorably moving interview with Harry Carpenter. 'I'm so delighted to have beaten a renowned champion so well,' Barry began, before adding, 'I'd like to take this opportunity to say one thing, and I've been thinking about it all week...' He took a deep breath to compose himself. He swallowed hard. 'I said if I won this world title I would dedicate it to a young lad that died when he fought me in 1982. I said at the start that I'd like it to be not just an ordinary fighter that beat him but a world champion...'

Barry desperately wanted to expand on this, say some more, perhaps even mention Young Ali by name, but it was no longer possible. Tears streamed down his face, his voice cracked and only the wide open arms of his father were able to console him.

'Barry McGuigan hugs his father, Pat, and he dedicates the fight to the young fighter who so tragically died after Barry had fought him some years ago,' concluded Carpenter.

THE RETURN

Three months after I stood beside Nick Blackwell's hospital bed and struggled to find the words to say to a boxer in a coma, I'm back covering fights at ringside. Chris Eubank Jr is back, too. He's on his way to the ring now, in fact, accompanied by the sounds of Dr Dre's 'Still Dre' and the presence of his father, still Chris Eubank. Some things never change. To quote an ageing, exasperated Michael Corleone, 'Just when I thought I was out... they pull me back in.' It speaks for so many of us.

This is not to say I ever intended to stay away from covering fights at ringside, nor stop watching them on television. But, certainly, a moralistic part of me liked to believe that all I'd heard, from the many fighters I'd interviewed for this book, and all I'd seen, while cooped up in St Mary's hospital, would at least provide me with some kind of cooling-off period, if not a complete denouncement of the sport. Alas, all the experience seemed to do, if I'm honest, is force me to first realise and then confess (to myself) just how much I really like watching human beings fight. Maybe even *love* watching human beings fight. It's a genuine source of enjoyment for me – violence done vicariously – and, without it, without this perverse pleasure, a significant part of me would be unsatisfied. Pro wrestling won't cut it. I'm aware of this now. I knew it the moment the next big fight came along and I was once again jonesing for drama, for action, for big punches, for a 'Fight of the Year' contender, in spite of all I'd seen and heard. I also knew that witnessing a friend in a coma, as a consequence of boxing, yet still wanting to watch the very thing that nearly killed him, can only be interpreted as a definitive mark of obsession.

We're all the same. Even Michael Watson in his auto-biography describes the WBC world super-middleweight title fight between Nigel Benn and Gerald McClellan on 25 February 1995 as 'one of the most amazing fights I have ever seen... which I know is probably impossible for many people to understand.' Impossible to understand because it was a bout that rendered McClellan totally blind, partially deaf and unable to walk unassisted, a bout that would damage the American worse than Eubank's eleventh round uppercut from hell damaged Watson. Yet it was also a bout Watson, four years on from his own near-tragedy, enjoyed from ringside.

I know this much: what happened to Nick Blackwell *did* change me as a spectator and altered the way I view boxing. That's unavoidable. If it hadn't, why else would I be so concerned for the well-being of Tom Doran, Chris Eubank Jr's next opponent, a man I've never met, before their fight at London's O2 Arena has even started? The Welshman seems overmatched and possesses a record that reveals he's not in the British champion's league. That concerns me. I am also concerned because I have come to understand Eubank Jr isn't exactly the forgiving type, nor is he anything like his father, at least not in this context. This means that for him, also, there will be no cooling-off period. There will be no introspection or self-doubt. The fact he injured Nick Blackwell three months ago counts for nothing right now. He has told us as much.

'I'm in there to win, defend myself and attack, and to further my career, so there is no mercy,' he said at a press conference in the days preceding the June fight. 'However cold that may sound, there is no mercy, no easing off. I have to go in there and be as ferocious as I can. It's the referee's job. It's not for me to have to say I should ease up. I've seen the consequences of what can happen when you're unprepared for a fight, or not as prepared as your opponent. I can't let anything like that happen to me. I've got too many goals, too much ambition.'

Across the room at the Canary Riverside Plaza Hotel, watching as his older brother addressed the media in a number of interviews, sat Sebastian Eubank, an amateur boxer in his own right, who moonlights as a personal trainer and spoken-word poet in his spare time. He was at the back of the room, towards the corner, happy to be out of sight – how very un-Eubank – and lowered his head in order to read messages on his phone and to enhance his anonymity. I was intrigued, both by the poetry and the eagerness to go unnoticed, so I went to gather some thoughts, some *considered* thoughts, on two men he knew better than perhaps anyone else.

'He was a very tunnel-vision kid,' is how Sebastian described his sibling. 'He'd focus on one thing at a time but put all his focus into it. I'm a bit more three-dimensional. I like to do a few different things rather than obsess over one.

Once Chris saw something, though, that was it. He wanted to do it and become the best at it.'

'Are you talking, specifically, about boxing?' I said.

'Yeah. He loves boxing. I don't really love boxing. I've just been around it so long, it's kind of become ingrained in me, whether it's my genetics or not. I can fight but he really loves to fight. He loves to do that more than anything else.

'Having him as an older brother meant we had our brotherly love scraps and he never held back. Even then he had that killer instinct in him. But that's what you need in boxing.'

The poet was never likely to have *it*. In that respect, he probably shared more of a kinship with his father than his brother. Gym rats used to tell me he was every bit as talented as his brother, but that didn't necessarily mean it was Sebastian's calling, nor did it mean he had the mindset for it. On the subject of mindsets, I asked him how his brother's might have changed given what happened to Nick Blackwell. The response was as definitive as it was obvious.

'I don't think it changed him whatsoever,' he said. 'We didn't find any fault. It's not on us. It's on them. My brother's job is to fight. We were trying to get it stopped earlier, but, if they're not going to do that, that's on them. Chris just went straight back to the gym after the fight. Obviously, we were worried for Nick while he was in hospital and were hoping he would recover, which he did, but, once he recovered, it was just a case of back to business.'

'He won't suffer the way your father did after Michael Watson...' I said.

Sebastian shook his head. 'The difference is what happened with Watson was a one-punch thing. It was just out of the blue, out of nowhere. I still think there are people who should be held accountable for what happened to Blackwell.

As far as Team Eubank are concerned, we just did our job. I don't think it's fair for Chris to take any blame for that. He was just in there fighting.'

'So, he'll be the same Chris on Saturday night...'

'If not even more ferocious. He wants a world title fight and he wants to prove a point and that means he's going to finish off any opponent he can get his hands on in the most devastating fashion.'

A mantra repeated by the entire Eubank family during fight week, the focus was clearly on driving forwards, forgetting the events of 26 March, and not falling victim to the post-tragedy mope that can consume and ruin even the most ruthlessly ambitious of men. 'Junior's not that sort of character,' Ronnie Davies told me. 'Chris, his dad, was very, very upset after Michael Watson. He couldn't get up for that first fight back. He boxed badly. I don't think he was ever the same. I could tell immediately. He was a more compassionate person. It played on his mind. Trust me, Junior ain't the same.'

On 1 February 1992, five months after the Michael Watson incident, Chris Eubank defended his WBO world super-middleweight title, the gold he acquired in beating Watson, against South African Thulani 'Sugar Boy' Malinga. There were six defeats to Malinga's name. He was tricky, a solid contender, and would go on to one day win a world championship of his own, but was unmistakably, at that particular time, an opponent Eubank was meant to defeat and look good doing so.

If only it were that simple. Eubank did win, even dropping Malinga in the fifth, but had to rely on a split-decision verdict after twelve rounds to retain his belt. He was subdued. There was no fire. He appeared disjointed, content to cruise, and the posing-to-punching ratio wasn't conducive to impressing onlookers, much less stopping Malinga within the scheduled distance. 'Good steady boxing,' was how Jim Watt described it in commentary, rather than the 'blood and thunder' the nation typically associated with Eubank. With thirty seconds to go, Eubank missed a right hand plucked straight from a cartoon, tripped over his own feet and fell on his face. There was some laughter and some boos and Eubank appeared happy to run laps of the ring for the remainder of the round, so content was he to go the distance and pick up the win in that manner.

Three days before his son returned to the ring following the injury of an opponent, I asked Eubank to sum up his showing against Malinga, as well as his entire post-Watson body of work. It was a question met with a frown, a pause and an index finger placed gently against his top lip. Naturally. Then he began to speak.

'It's not that I lost anything,' he said, taking umbrage with the idea of depletion in light of the fact he went on to defend his WBO world super-middleweight title some fourteen times. 'I was benevolent. I was kind. I'm a kind spirit. I'm not there to take the spirit out of the man's mother. I'm not there to squash and desolate her spirit. I'm there to score more points than the man and beat him over a period of rounds. If I should damage him, it should only be for ten seconds and no more. To do that to a man's mother was hurtful to my spirit because my spirit is kind. I didn't want to do that to his mother. *I* have a mother.'

Michael Watson changed Chris Eubank, that is beyond dispute, but Michael Watson also changed British boxing and, for that, so many owe him a debt of gratitude. Nick Blackwell is just one example of someone who may not be alive today if it wasn't for the many changes the sport had to undergo as a result of what happened to Watson at White Hart Lane in 1991. Count them up. Paramedics on standby? Check.

Oxygen at ringside? Check. Prepped ambulances ready to take boxers to a designated hospital which specialises in injuries to the brain? Check. Neurological hospital within a ten-minute radius of the arena? Check. All of these things were introduced due to the backlash boxing received in the aftermath of a WBO world super-middleweight title fight watched by thirteen million people on ITV. They were introduced because Michael Watson fought for them to be introduced.

Indeed, much like his fighting style, Watson was headstrong and persistent. In September 1994 he sued the British Boxing Board of Control for negligence and eight years after the fight the High Court found them to have been negligent in not providing appropriate resuscitation equipment at ringside and doctors properly qualified to use it. The board was instructed to pay Watson damages and ended up selling their London headquarters in order to do so. Mr Justice Kennedy said the board was 'in breach of its duty to Mr Watson'. Mr Watson and so many others.

Also in the nineties, hot on the heels of two tragedies involving first Bradley Stone (1994) and then James Murray (1995), promoter Frank Warren wrote a cheque for £400,000 to set up the Murray Stone Fund, which would finance Magnetic Resonance Imaging (MRI) scans, more revealing than Computerised Tomography (CT) scans, for every professional boxer in Britain (approximately eight hundred at the time). The typical cost of an MRI scan was around £500 and Warren's Murray Stone Fund allowed boxers the luxury of drawing from the fund to ensure they received the most stringent tests. 'I'm being realistic,' said Warren. 'I don't think there's a lot you can do regarding death and what happens in the ring. There are tragedies in the sport, as indeed there are tragedies in other sports. As promoters, we feel we have a responsibility. We want to put something back into the sport and help the boxers.'

The only ones who didn't benefit from these wholesale changes were the fallen and perhaps the ones unfairly deemed responsible. For instance, Drew Docherty, the Scotsman who knocked out James Murray on that fateful night (13 October 1995) in Glasgow to retain the British bantamweight title, politely declined to be interviewed for this book because, and I quote, 'I am not talking about a tragedy in my life that was very hard to get over. To bring all the sadness and bad memories of that night back is too much. Even telling you this is bringing memories back – sadness I thought I had got over.'

No amount of after-the-fact rule changes or safety precautions could soothe *his* pain. I felt dirty for even breaching the subject.

Liverpool's Richie Wenton, though, did agree to meet me. He knocked out Bradley Stone in round ten of a British super-bantamweight title fight at York Hall, Bethnal Green on 26 April 1994, but remembers only 'four or five' of the rounds they shared, so traumatised was he by the experience. 'That fight devastated my reputation,' he said to me in a Sheffield pub. 'It wasn't like what happened to Barry McGuigan [who, incidentally, called Wenton after the Stone incident to offer his support]. A similar thing happened to him but he was able to move on. Why? Maybe because it was early in his career and he was up against a fella from Africa. I don't know. But my tragedy happened in a title fight against a British guy from London, so the whole situation was different. They wanted to crucify someone for what happened. They needed to hold someone responsible for it.'

Boxing, he feels, almost damaged him beyond repair. It ended the life of Bradley Stone, which, in turn, ruined his own chances of ever becoming a world champion, it painted him as a 'murderer' in the eyes of the British public, and it also impacted him in ways he'd only come to realise and understand once retired at thirty-three and pursuing a career as an offshore electrician.

'Sometimes I'd finish sparring at the gym and start to wonder about the damage punches were doing to me,' said Richie. 'There was definitely something in my mind after the Bradley Stone fight. I never used to have those thoughts after sparring, but sparring does more damage to a fighter than anything else. You see fighters out there now who can barely talk properly and a lot of that is because of the thousands of rounds they did in sparring. Boxing's a fucking dangerous sport, mate. I know that now. Don't get me wrong, it's one of the best sports in the world to watch, but it's so, so dangerous. I'd never put any of my children in boxing. I'd rather they played football. I'm lucky, I got out at the right time. My memory isn't great – I forget little things – but I'm not at the stage where I'm forgetting names or faces.'

Wenton showed no aversion to talking. Over a large cappuccino, he spoke at length about his upbringing, about the time he watched his father murder his mother on Boxing Day in 1972, about later living with his unstable father, about the message his father scrawled on the white walls of their Lodge Lane home – 'There is No Evil in This House' – and about how he had no choice but to then follow in his father's footsteps in becoming a boxer. He also, of course, spoke about Bradley Stone, and about his first fight after the tragedy, a non-title bout with Neil Swain in which he turned his back on his opponent in round five and refused to fight any more, basically surrendering, to the disbelief of all those who had watched him dominate the bout. 'I wasn't afraid of getting hurt after the Bradley Stone fight, but I was afraid that someone else could get hurt,' he explained. 'I was terrified of it happening again.'

One thing Wenton won't do, however, is contemplate returning to York Hall, the scene of the so-called crime, a place he still adores and calls 'the home of boxing'. It is simply off-limits, he stressed, and has been ever since that nightmarish incident in 1994. 'I've seen it on television plenty of times, and that's okay, but I'd never want to go into the hall itself. It's a shame, too, because I had the happiest day of my life in that place. But I'll never go there again.'

It's the reticence of the former fighter that stays with you above everything else. Some verbalise it and tell you point-blank their trauma is a no-go area, while for others it's written all over their face. Irrespective of how it's projected, the feeling it generates sticks. Or at least it did with me. For me this journey would merely culminate in some kind of story, maybe a lesson, yet for them, those tragic characters sprinkled throughout, the story was all too real. It could be viewed a bit like a fight, I suppose. A fight, after all, is one thing to us – the spectator, the peanut gallery embracing the perks of distance and disconnect – and something else entirely in the minds of those involved, namely the fighters. To us, it is entertainment, a night out. To them, it truly is a matter of life or death. And what's entertaining about that?

Back at the O2 Arena, Tom Doran, Chris Eubank Jr's opponent, nay, sacrificial lamb, is doing far better than many anticipated, meaning he has made it through the first two rounds, landed some cute counter hooks of his own, and so far avoided becoming the man against whom Eubank Jr intends to prove a point. But, in round three, things quickly unravel. He is momentarily paralysed by a left hook to the body, which is followed by a right round the other side, and then driven towards the ropes as the crowd rise to their feet and clap and cheer and shout and roar. This is what they came for, and Eubank Jr acts on this hunger. There's no let-up. Four more punches follow, including a right uppercut, as the noise around him intensifies. Seven more go in, thrown mostly to the body, before another uppercut lands, cracks Doran's nose and he drops to the canvas on his knees. Scent of knockout strong, Eubank Jr retreats to a neutral corner and turns to face the baying audience. His eyes blacken, he's barely breathing, and he seems to delight in being able to give us all what we want.

Poor Tom Doran. He beats the count, but rounds one and two, rounds in which he competed on an even keel, are now a distant memory. As a right to the body folds him again in the fourth, and another right uppercut downs him moments later, a woman with an Essex twang, sat directly behind me, becomes wise to what is unfolding and says to her friend, 'He's going to get hurt, that kid.'

She's right.

A final uppercut, thrown as Doran looks to escape to the neutral corner, completes the job. 'Stop the fight!' cries the woman behind me. Luckily, the referee, Marcus McDonnell, does just that, after which Eubank Jr raises a fist in celebration and Doran, as brave as he was outclassed, stumbles back to his corner, sits down on the stool and sucks up air from an oxygen mask passed to him by the ringside doctor.

For a moment, I panic and wonder, will it now always be this way?

Two weeks after I watch Chris Eubank Jr return to the ring, Dan Blackwell, Nick's younger brother, fights two-bout novice Luke Heron over four rounds at the Town Hall in Walsall.

Yeah, you guessed it. He too was unable to stay away.

Put in context, Blackwell's defeat to Heron would be the fifty-fifth of his professional career, but he lost only by a point and, crucially, received little damage in the process. It was, therefore, in the eyes of Dan Blackwell, the journeyman, a job well done, one worthy of a dramatic U-turn.

So long as they are all like this – close losses, little in the way of pain – it seems only natural he will continue boxing for a number of years. He is still young. There is still money to be made alongside his full-time work as a bricklayer, and a young family to support. He also now has the blessing of Nick and has been training alongside him in Trowbridge. They've been running together, doing pads together, even sparring together, though Dan is quick to emphasise it's only 'body sparring', whereby head shots are strictly prohibited.

'What you're doing is totally different to what I was doing,' Nick told him. 'You're only doing four and six rounds and you know how to protect yourself. You don't get hit as much as I did. Just get back in there.'

Often it's the winning, or at least the pursuit of victory, that gets a fighter hurt. It leaves them susceptible to getting hit, getting punished, *not winning*. Dan strives to be competitive whenever he fights, pride ensures that, but he doesn't always seek the win. A win to him is a far simpler concept. A win to him is making it through the scheduled four or six rounds, teaching his novice opponent a thing or two along the way, and, most importantly, getting out unscathed, thus being fit to fight again soon after. It's why, at just twenty-three years of age, he already has sixty-two fights to his name, and it's why Nick, his brother, someone forced to stop boxing because of its dangers, gives him the two thumbs up to continue.

THE HAPPY
ENDING

Six months on from what he now calls the best sleep of his life, otherwise known as an induced coma, Nick Blackwell has boxing gloves on his hands, stands in an orthodox fighting stance, left foot forward, right foot back, and receives hooked punches to his head from a much bigger, tattooed brute. The blows are only light, I hasten to add, and the idea is to block them before they connect, but some get through, causing his head to rattle on impact, and I'm shocked by the scene which greets me upon entering the Fight Science gym in Aldershot's military barracks.

Immediately I want to yell out for them both to 'Stop!' the way my mother would whenever she caught me and my brothers midway through pillow fights in the living room. Rather than concerned about the possibility of a light bulb being cracked, a mirror being smashed or the television being upended, I am instead worried about a boxer going to sleep again – and for longer this time.

Feeling enlightened, I have an urge to share tales of Al Seeger's nose bleeds and Frankie Leal's desire to keep fighting following a head injury. So I sit on a wooden bench and wait for my moment. I watch Nick take young offenders and victims of bullying on the pads. I watch him have fun and enjoy himself, all for a good cause. Then, when it's time for a well-earned lunch break, he joins me on the bench, seems happy to spot a familiar face, and thanks me for returning to my hometown to visit him.

Screw pleasantries, I think. Get straight down to it. 'I didn't expect you to be getting hit around the head,' I say, coming over all parental.

He laughs. 'Oh, that's nothing. I had my first sparring session on Monday.'

Gulp. 'Full-on sparring?' I say.

'Yeah. We only did a few rounds but I felt good. Well, I felt like shit – I'm so unfit – but it was fine. I took a few shots.'

Seven days of slumber led to months of rehabilitation but Nick was right. He was fine. One of the lucky ones. Made a full recovery. A quick one at that. But, such is the drive of the high-performance athlete, he wanted it to be quicker. In hospital, he told nurses he wanted to walk, so he walked, unsteadily at first, and then he told them he wanted to do one hundred press-ups, a feat he achieved with ease before his accident, only to give it a go and manage six. The next day he hit sixteen. By the end of the week he was at sixty-five. This, in many ways, summarised his recovery: initial enthusiasm and impatience getting the better of him, but steady improvements made on a daily basis.

The mind was a tougher opponent to master. Blackwell

was a fit, strong athlete, albeit one who plummeted to nine-and-a-half stone while bed-bound, and was expected to soon excel again physically, yet the mind, he discovered, doesn't care much for six-packs or biceps. For a while it deceived him. It played tricks on him. There were pictures of giraffes flashed before his eyes and when asked to specify if what he saw depicted was a cat, a dog or, you guessed it, a giraffe, Blackwell for a while was convinced what he saw on the card was a cat. 'My head was that bad,' he says. 'I couldn't take anything in. I didn't know what I was doing. The doctor said to my family, "That's probably the best he's ever going to be." Imagine what it was like for them.'

He asked his father, John, to get him some word-search puzzles and so began the process of re-training his mind, training it just as he'd once trained his body before fights. It would take a couple of months to right itself – poor memory and concentration were obstacles he had to overcome – but, certainly, sitting beside him now, watching him prise a sandwich from cellophane, I sense no hangover from the events of March. He's just as lucid as before the fight, if not more so, for now he's enhanced by a kind of awakening and appreciation of life that can only be unlocked when cheating death, and his sense of humour remains, if now an even darker shade of black.

'You got any bouts lined up, Nick?' asks one of the men sweating, wraps on hands, having just completed a workout in the gym.

I want to hide. I glance over at Nick, hoping he isn't in some way insulted or embarrassed, and find a man straight-faced and hard-to-read. 'Yeah,' he says. 'It's looking like December the fifteenth for my next one.'

I frown but say nothing.

'Oh, yeah?' says the man. 'Where will that be?'

'Manchester.'

'That's great. Who will you be fighting?'

'Eubank,' says Nick, still appearing to be serious. 'We're doing the rematch. Time to get my revenge.'

'Even better. God, I'd love to see you smash him. He needs a good humbling, that kid.'

Another man overhears the conversation and can't help but interject. 'I thought they said you couldn't box again,' he says.

Nick's grin gives the game away. 'You're right. I can't. I'm only joking, guys.'

The men laugh about it. Nick does the same. But then one of them gets serious and says, 'Did the doctors say for certain you can't box?'

'Well, no,' replies Nick, 'but I'd be in a high-risk category. It's not worth it.'

'Shame. I'd have loved to see you beat that Eubank kid. Did you read what he said the other day about Kell Brook?'

Five days ago, Kell Brook, Britain's IBF world welterweight champion, audaciously moved up two weight classes to face IBF and WBC world middleweight champion Gennady Golovkin of Kazakhstan and received a broken orbital bone and a fifth-round stoppage, the first loss of his professional career, for his troubles. He also suffered the indignity of having Chris Eubank Jr, the natural middleweight originally lined up to fight Golovkin at London's O2 Arena, make light of the anti-climactic way in which he lost, which is to say he criticised Brook's coach and cornerman, Dominic Ingle, for compassionately waving the white towel in round five, thus saving his fighter. For some reason, Eubank Jr, taking to Twitter immediately after the fight, was having none of it. He wrote: 'Gennady Golovkin, if you want a fight with a real British middleweight... come get some. My corner don't own towels.' The Eubank Jr view was that Brook's corner had realised their man was out of his depth and cut the night short when the going got tough. But very few agreed with this line of thinking. Nor did it hold too much weight given it was Eubank Jr who turned down a fight with Golovkin on 10 September, only for Brook to take the same deal and fill the void.

Even so, the next day, in an interview on Sky Sports News, the Eubanks, Junior *and* Senior, attempted to explain what was meant by the message. 'It wasn't meant to disrespect anybody,' said Junior. 'It's just how I've been brought up, how I've been taught as a fighter. You don't look for your corner to end the fight. The only person who is supposed to be stopping the fight is the referee. The corner is there to clean your cuts up and put your Vaseline on, not throw in the towel. If the going gets tough, you stay in there and take your beating like a man...' His father, stood to his left in a black shirt buttoned to the top and holding a Louis Vuitton man-bag beneath his left arm, nodded his head approvingly. 'That's what we sign up for.'

'That's right,' said Senior.

'That's all that was meant when I said my corner don't own towels. They would never throw in the towel. They'd let me try and win and get myself out of a sticky situation. Just because you're getting hurt doesn't mean you can't come back and win.'

'It's the hurt business and that's what we're in it for – to persevere,' added Senior. 'You cannot expect to get anywhere near greatness if you're not prepared to accept damage. We are not fans, we are doing it. You are not like us, you don't think like us. Hurt is good. Damage is good. We have to be that way. We cannot be like, "Oh, I'm getting hurt, so I'm going to quit." You can't make greatness like that. The language of a warrior is, "I'm going to go all the way."'

Thanks to the countless contradictions which emerged during this latest pursuit of publicity, it was becoming tougher and tougher to defend the Eubanks, let alone buy into the father's theory that he helped save the life of Nick Blackwell on 26 March. There were too many crossed wires and things which didn't add up.

Yet here's what I do know. I know Chris Eubank didn't rewrite history. He wasn't aware of the developing narrative when he told me, half an hour after the fight, that he'd deliberately made a point of instructing his son to target his opponent's body. Nor was he pandering to any great audience – there was none. He didn't mention the moment to anoint himself a lifesaver or reveal the depths of his compassion and he didn't relay the information with any great deal of pride, either. He merely used it as an example of how one-sided they, Team Eubank, perceived the fight to have become.

I also refuse to believe that the call for his son to target Nick Blackwell's body was *solely* tactical. Not after speaking to him beforehand and then in the changing room and not after spending twelve months conversing with men who admitted to being scarred and changed by the trauma of seeing an opponent meet their end. No, to classify Chris Eubank's corner monologue as merely tactical, when the punches were hurtful and faces were disfigured, is to surely disregard his thirteen-year professional boxing career – all those punches, all those concussions, all those memories – and the very thing that altered him in 1991. Sure, you and I and every armchair coach in the land might instruct a boxer to target the body when the head seems carved from granite – for it's the done thing, it's obvious – but do the considered (sometimes *too* considered) words of Eubank not hold more weight? Do they not come from a deeper and darker place? Of course they do. I'd even go as far as to argue Eubank's understanding of boxing is greater than many of his peers, and I say this because he is well versed in the extremes. He has experienced the very best and the very worst, whereas the majority of boxers, those spared tragedy in the ring, are unable to say the same. Their lowest point, a surprising defeat, let's say, or the loss of a world title, cannot possibly compare to the horror of seeing an opponent slip to the canvas and be removed from the ring on a stretcher, later to be determined either dead or in some way incapacitated.

Moreover, Michael Watson, unlike the deceased opponents of those boxers featured in this book, never leaves Eubank. He miraculously survived. He lives on. He's omnipresent. His name is still relevant, spoken and celebrated, and it has been this way for a quarter of a century. There are constant reminders wherever Eubank goes. Still attached to the 'mug's game', there are reminders in the gym, when overseeing his son prepare for battle, there are reminders at press conferences, when hearing his son engage in trash talk with an opponent, and there are reminders on fight night, when his son attempts to violently back up his boasts and render someone unconscious. It's highly unlikely, therefore, that the memories mysteriously dried up at the crucial moment his son, having landed an obscene amount of uppercuts (the Watson shot) on the jaw of his opponent, returned to the corner at the end of round eight on 26 March 2016.

Blackwell, it must be said, never subscribed to this theory.

He knew his life wasn't saved by Chris Eubank and he knew the call to target his body wasn't made with his well-being in mind. It was a stance many shared, especially those within the fight game, and I too could certainly see how the call was interpreted this way – as strategy. It is, after all, a command followers of boxing frequently hear whenever a television microphone is placed near a boxer's corner in between rounds. The words are so commonplace they hardly register, until something awful happens. I could also understand the scepticism of those who felt it behooved Eubank to manipulate the narrative upon realising the uneducated masses mistook strategic instructions for a compassionate plea and thus heralded him a saviour. It's an easy assumption to make because Eubank has always coveted attention, publicity, the limelight, the director's chair.

But that was six months ago. Now, with a fresh Eubank riddle to solve, one inspired by Kell Brook and a white towel, it was impossible to feel strongly one way or another. Think about it. On one hand, father and son claimed boxers needed to be protected from damage and from themselves, yet on the other hand, a revised theory announced to the world six months after the Blackwell incident, they suggested boxers should fight until they are no longer able to. Ignore damage. Ignore your corner. Ignore it all if you want to become great. Hmmm. Whether the bravado and bluster of narcissists, the holier-than-thou but ultimately mumbo-jumbo of men who overstate their intelligence, or simply an indication of how paradoxical the sport of boxing can be, how mixed its message can be, the Eubank preaching had well and truly run its course by September.

The soldiers in Aldershot agree. They roll their eyes. One even points at a poster on the gym wall of Michael Watson, set to fight Nigel Benn in 1989, and says, 'Eubank should bloody know better. He should keep his mouth shut.'

Blackwell, for his part, has chosen to do just that. He no longer wants to speak about either Eubank, nor does he like reflecting on the way they behaved in the aftermath of their March fight. He has said enough, he believes. Too much, if anything. His exclusive in the *Sun*, in which he allegedly said he'd like to land a final punch on Chris Eubank's jaw, did far more harm than good, and the same can be said for his appearance on *Good Morning Britain*, which is also now a cause of embarrassment and regret. 'I was badly advised,' he says, 'and it was too soon.'

So badly advised was Blackwell that an inbox full of well-wishers turned to one full of trolls lambasting him for turning on the Eubanks and being 'bitter' about what happened to him. They said he should instead be thanking the Eubanks for their class, their dignity and their compassion. His price to pay, Nick defended himself and proclaimed innocence, as was his right, but it didn't take long for him to realise he'd gone the wrong way about explaining what he believed to be salient points; perhaps, in hindsight, his mind wasn't yet ready to properly connect with his mouth in order to articulate not only his own thought process but also the agenda imprinted on him by others ('The Eubanks are bad, Nick, they're evil, Nick, they said this and they did that while you were in a coma, Nick'). The backlash hurt. It saddened him. He temporarily closed his social media accounts.

Still, nothing depresses Blackwell quite like the feeling of being unfit. Holidays, two of them back-to-back, saw him reach a lifetime-heaviest thirteen stone six in recent weeks. 'Thirteen stone,' he says, standing on a set of scales by the gym entrance. 'I've lost some of it, but nowhere near enough.' This aspect, the lack of abdominals, seems to bother Blackwell more than it would most. It's on his mind as we leave the gym and it's on his mind when a chubby boy in a Ralph Lauren polo shirt asks him if he intends on fighting again. 'Yeah,' says Nick, 'as a heavyweight.' The boy laughs. It's also on his mind when Nick later opens the boot of his car and switches his damp workout T-shirt for a fresher one, only after pinching his bare midriff and sides. 'People think I'm mad,' he says. 'They go, "You're fine, Nick, you still look in good shape." But they don't understand. I've *never* been this fat. When I sit down there's a ripple of fat on my belly that has never been there before.'

I want to join the club and say, 'You're fine, Nick, you still look in good shape,' but decide against it. We're in an underground car park. He's topless. There are people within earshot. It feels weird. I say nothing. He changes his top, closes his car boot and we move on. 'I'm going to get really fit again,' he mutters, as if to motivate himself. 'Fitter than I ever was when I was fighting.' I believe him.

When we reach Caffe Macchiato in Aldershot town centre he orders a latte and enquires about fruit. He asks the girl behind the counter if she has any – a request denied – before explaining, 'I always get a craving for some cake after a coffee. Fruit is a good substitute.' Evidently, he wants to lead by example. He wants to eat clean. He also wants to start reading books. It's something foreign to him, he informs me, something that hadn't previously fit into his routine, but he wants to change that now. In a show of intent, I recommended *Barbarian Days: A Surfing Life* by William Finnegan a couple of days ago and he immediately jumped into his car and raced to the nearest book shop in Trowbridge to find a copy. 'I need to work my brain more,' he explains. 'It's a muscle like anything else. Boxing, the routine, the punches, it dumbs you down. I want to grow as a human being now.'

He also wants to surf. He wants to do *that* more than anything. And he got the chance to finally do so back in July when he travelled to Cornwall in his VW Transporter with his best friend Jake, and indulged in some surfing and coasteering and then recklessly plummeted off rocks from a height of somewhere around forty feet. Totally against doctor's orders, Nick stuck to his plan regardless. This was, he imagined, the fun bit, the brief interlude between a boxing life and a working life, one he hoped to eventually turn into a surfing life. What that constitutes, I'm not entirely sure, but Nick's long-term goal, once his tan began to fade, his waistline started to expand and the banality of civilian life resumed, was to use the money he made from boxing, as well as the money received from fundraisers, to set up a gym and health cafe in Trowbridge.

Up on the rocks, though, he was just happy to have made a full recovery and to be set free. He would make no apology for it, either, and was quick to call what happened in March a 'blessing in disguise', if only because it provided him with a clearly signposted exit and a new lease of life. He says he can live like a normal human being now, following years of rigorous training and dieting and being starved of such simple pleasures as socialising, holidaying and eating, and feels no sentimentality towards boxing, his former love. 'The whole game is corrupt,' he tells me. 'It's more of a business than a sport. It's a mug's game.'

Now emancipated, as he walked the Pentire headland and flung himself forty feet from a rock and aimed to hit the water before hitting something else, namely another rock,

Blackwell wasn't thinking about this 'mug's game' or his next opponent or his regimented calorie intake or a training circuit or a sparring session he had to endure later that day. He wasn't thinking about any of that stuff because it had all become irrelevant. Instead, he thought about purer pursuits, like surfing. He thought about a life without boxing. He thought about the thrill of being able to drive again, having been temporarily prevented from doing so, and the places he and his friend would visit next. He thought about the possibility of his friend cracking his head on a rock if he dared to get any closer to the one he'd just narrowly avoided. He thought about buying properties. He thought about his new gym. He thought about the boxers at his old gym, such as Enzo Maccarinelli, Liam Williams, Alex Hughes and Dale Evans, and their trainer, Gary Lockett, who he still visits and trains alongside from time to time. He thought about the sacrifices they all still have to make. He thought about the damage boxing has yet to do to them. They might have it coming, he thought. He then thought how lucky he has been to have escaped now, at twenty-five, with relatively few miles on the clock and relatively few scars on his face.

Maybe, in the end, he *has* to think like this because it's the easiest way of coping and moving on. But, maybe, just maybe, he has been truly enlightened and it's Nick Blackwell, more than anyone else featured in this book, who has inadvertently found himself on the path to some kind of salvation.

One thing I *do* know is that day in Cornwall there wasn't a single thought spared for the possibility of him banging his head. 'I just love that fear that you might hurt yourself,' he says. 'I'm surprised I didn't die.'

THE HAPPY ENDING

Ring, ring.

He didn't know it at the time but this was to be the phone call that changed George Khalid Jones' life, or, as he puts it, elevated him to a higher place. It was, ironically enough, a phone call his wife, Naomi, had been threatening to make for weeks. But each time she punched in the number, heard the dial tone and then detected the voice of a female on the other end she just as quickly cut off the call and dropped the phone. Took a deep breath. Controlled her racing heartbeat. Collected her thoughts. Told her husband she just couldn't do it.

Then one day, owing to either woman's intuition or sheer dumb luck, Denise Scottland, the intended recipient, got the message and succeeded where Naomi failed. She grabbed the phone, dialled the Jones residence and asked to speak with Khalid. Her opening words were simple yet profound: 'I don't blame you.'

George Khalid Jones had knocked out Denise's twenty-six-year-old husband, Beethavean 'Bee' Scottland, with just thirty-seven seconds left in a light-heavyweight boxing match on the deck of the USS *Intrepid*, New York, on 26 June 2001. Before the Tuesday night bout he had said, 'I trained so hard, I'm afraid I'm going to kill somebody.' Six days later, at 10:36p.m. on the evening of 2 July 2001, Jones' premonition came true. Bee Scottland was pronounced dead of a subdural haematoma, a rupture of the veins between the brain and the skull.

Khalid, a broken, remorseful man, attended Bee's funeral, announced his intentions to quit the sport, returned to his full-time job as an inventory specialist at a Paterson printing shop, and found close allies in Hennessy and Heineken. His routine became a destructive one. Most mornings he woke, brushed his teeth and stared in the mirror, only to then return to bed for the rest of the day. The bed cover went all the way over his head. Sometimes he'd sob, other times he'd just be silent.

It wasn't until the phone rang one day that all this changed.

'It was only when Denise called me and told me not to retire that I changed my mind,' said Khalid. 'Denise made me realise there's nothing wrong with forgiving or accepting something. She said it wasn't my fault and that her husband wouldn't be angry with me right now.'

In awe of the strength of the woman, Khalid acquiesced. He returned to the ring in December of 2001 in a fight against Philadelphian southpaw Eric Harding. But it was easier said than done. 'I used to train like I wanted to kill somebody, like I knew they were going to go down,' Khalid said. 'I tried to punch *through* my opponent. But after what happened to Bee, I didn't want to hurt anyone no more. I just wanted to win fights without hurting anyone. I didn't want to kill anybody. I'm not a murderer. If you'd have caught me twenty-five years ago on the street, I'd have been like, "If they do wrong, they've got to die." That was my way of thinking. But that was a lifetime ago. Now I was scared for my opponent and myself. Now I told my trainer, "I don't want to die in there. Don't let me die in there. You have to know when to stop it."'

A week before the fight, Khalid broke down in tears during a television interview. He admitted feeling 'compassion' for the first time in his career. Those around him were flabbergasted. *Compassion*? For a fighter, it was the absolute worst thing to feel before a fight.

That wasn't all. On fight night, Jones, with 'Bee' and 'RIP' emblazoned on his fight shorts, hit Harding, his opponent, with a decent shot, only to then back away. He did so out of fear. Johnny Bos, the matchmaker sat at ringside, shook his head. His biggest concern had become a reality.

Didn't take long for Harding to come to this realisation, either. He dominated the contest, hurt Khalid in the sixth round and then finished him in the seventh with a seven-punch combination. Jones, out of his depth, slid to the canvas as his wife Naomi and eleven-year-old daughter Aisha cried uncontrollably at ringside. It was over. The fight, his career, everything. Bos told him so afterwards.

It wasn't, of course. A boxer's career rarely ends when it should. There would be more fights, more defeats, more punches to the head and body. Wins, too, but never enough to bag the world title shot he craved. That failed to materialise no matter how hard he tried.

In the end, Khalid made do. He faced Darnell 'Ding-A-Ling Man' Wilson on 3 August 2004 with something far greater than a world title at stake. A routine ten-rounder on paper, that night in Glen Burnie, Maryland, Denise Scottland made the trip and would sit ringside to support Jones. Denise cheered, applauded and inspired Jones to a hard-fought draw. She implored him to 'hold on' when he was hurt. She whooped and hollered every punch he threw in response. It was, to her, just like the old days, no different to when she used to encourage Bee from ringside. 'It's something I've talked about with Naomi,' Denise told the *Baltimore Sun*. 'I used to tell Bee that I was his number-one fan. Now, Naomi is Khalid's number-one fan. But I'm his number-two fan.'

Bee Scottland was one of eight children born to a corrections officer and a classical pianist and grew up in Brentwood, a low-income suburb of Washington, DC. Life there had been tough for him – not Khalid tough, but tough enough. He supplemented his stop–start boxing career with work as an exterminator, so keen was he to provide for Denise and their eight-year-old daughter and two sons aged six and two, and had learnt to appreciate the simple things in life. The $7,000 he got for facing Jones in New York was the biggest payday of his six-year professional boxing career. Jones, in many ways, could relate. 'We both wanted the same thing,' he said. 'A shot at something better.'

Jones, wrecked by a recurring back injury, retired from boxing in 2005. His family send gifts to the Scottlands every Christmas, despite not celebrating the festive period themselves, and Khalid still regularly speaks to Denise, his 'angel', his 'little sister', on the phone. He has even promised to pay her kids' college tuition fees and reminds her of this near enough every time they communicate.

Little Bee, the youngest of Denise's children, is never far from Khalid's mind. He's fifteen now and has grown up without a father. Khalid knows the importance of having one of those. Still, the kid's doing okay. Recently Khalid, a father of five, was told Little Bee was again trying out for the school basketball team having been unsuccessful in his attempt the previous year.

'Why didn't it work out for you last year?' Khalid asked him over the phone.

'Coach said I wasn't good enough,' said Little Bee.

Khalid shook his head. 'Okay,' he said, 'Who's your favourite player?'

'Kevin Durant,' replied Little Bee, certain of it.

'Right, I'll tell you what, if you make the team, I'll get you some Kevin Durant sneakers and will deliver them to your house,' said Khalid, whose business, Champ's Trucking, is a freight delivery service, and whose favourite NBA player also happened to be the then-Oklahoma City Thunder small forward.

Little Bee missed out on making the team for a second year, but it didn't matter. He was still consoled by the sight of a pair of Kevin Durant sneakers and socks mailed to his house by the Joneses.

'You didn't have to do this,' Little Bee said, having raced to the phone to tell Khalid all about the package. 'I didn't even make the team.'

'That don't matter,' said Khalid. 'I believe players can motivate kids. Durant is a great player. Go be like him.'

'I will.'

'So, anyway, how do you like the sneakers?'

'I don't like them.'

'Oh.'

'I *love* them.'

THE END

THE END

Sometimes I wonder how difficult it would be discussing this book's subject matter with an active boxer, particularly a boxer not yet affected by the death or serious injury of an opponent. My guess is it would be akin to showing a Formula One driver videos of car crashes and mangled motors just before they hit the starting grid, or showing an American football player scans of CTE-afflicted brains, or simply showing an obese adult the true content of their Happy Meal. Insensitive at best, life-changing at worst, the boxer's response would serve as a reminder that no man or woman wants to confront the harsh reality of boxing while still calling it their livelihood. There'd be questions. An abundance of them. Some might be spoken out loud, but most would be internalised. And that's where the real problem lies. Picture it. Inquisitive boxer discovers the testimonies of those featured in this book only to then stew on it, freak out and finally reassess the virtues of a martial art they have practised and relied upon since childhood. Like a meat-eater turning vegetarian, this leads to a moment of clarity – eureka! – and then an abrupt retirement. It's the outcome that frightens me. Too much power, responsibility and guilt on my part. It's unwelcome. I'm not here to preach or show prizefighters a road to salvation. How hypocritical. Truth is, I'm every bit as obsessed with violence, and, some would say, in need of saving, as they are. So don't listen to me, I want to say, and please don't read this. Just see for yourself.

To avoid this conversation, I draw up an imaginary non-disclosure agreement with the fight fraternity: for eighteen months, I'll say nothing. When in the company of active boxers I consider friends, those with whom I communicate on a semi-regular basis, I'll say nothing. Nothing about the book, nothing about its subject matter. It's better this way, safer this way. It's for your own good, I'll tell them.

One Wednesday in November, however, George Groves, an active boxer, gets wind of something brewing and proceeds to shatter our agreement, one to which he is oblivious, as I'm cornered in the kitchen area of his Hammersmith boxing gym sipping tap water from a Chelsea Football Club mug and he's lacing his boxing boots ahead of a sparring session, his last before a fight in nine days. There was, in retrospect, no worse time for our discussion to unfold.

'So,' he says, 'I hear you're writing a book.'

'Yes,' I reply, sheepishly, swig of water used to break eye contact. 'I am.'

'What's it about?'

'I'm not really comfortable telling you, to be honest,' I mumble. 'Not when you're just about to spar. Not when you have a fight coming up.'

'What do you mean?'

THE END

'Well, it's about boxers who have "killed",' I make quotation marks with the index and middle finger of both hands, 'opponents in the ring.'

'Oh, right. That's dark.'

'You can see why I didn't want to tell you.'

He shrugs. 'Do you know who you are going to interview for it?'

'The book's done.'

'Really? You never even mentioned you were writing it.'

'I know.'

'Have you included any stuff from this year or is it more historical?'

'A bit of both. It was supposed to be historical, but Nick Blackwell's injury at Wembley was the first I'd seen in person.'

'Yeah, that wasn't nice.'

'Did you know he was concussed before that fight?'

'Yeah. He came down here a few times before the fight and the last time we sparred...'

'I was here.'

'Oh, yeah. I forgot.' George fetches some hand wraps. 'I heard he wasn't right after we sparred. It's so dangerous going through with a fight if you ain't feeling well. That's a different type of injury to a fucked-up hand. You can't risk it.'

Exactly a fortnight after I checked on Nick Blackwell in Aldershot and found a twenty-five-year-old fortunate to still be alive and now embracing all life has to offer, another twenty-five-year-old, Mike Towell, required a stretcher to depart a boxing ring in Glasgow following a fifth-round knockout defeat, the first of his career. Twenty-four hours later, on the Friday, the very same day I happened to visit the Peacock Gym in Canning Town and gaze at the bronze Bradley Stone memorial statue located outside its entrance,

Towell tragically passed away. There were reports of chronic headaches in training, warning signs, worrying signs, but 'Iron' Mike, one of many who surrender to the same code, needed a fight and the money it would bring. He left behind a partner, Chloe, and a two-year-old son, Rocco.

Towell's opponent, meanwhile, was twenty-four-year-old Dale Evans, a Welsh gymmate of Nick Blackwell, who visited Nick at St Mary's Hospital in April. Welterweight Evans, like Towell, knew the dangers of his chosen profession – he'd recently witnessed its wrath first-hand – but never did he think tragedy would impact him, never did he think he'd be inextricably tied to a deceased boxer, never did he think he'd all of a sudden be infamous, and never did he think, days after it happening, a tragedy now headline news, he'd start to get the messages and the phone calls and the questions. 'So, Dale, how do you feel?'

Nobody expects it to happen to them. That's why, when it does, the metaphorical sucker punch catches them cold and turns their legs to jelly and their brains to mush. It's this very innocence that allows these men and women to fight in the first place; this ignorance, this delusion, this ill-judged sense of invincibility. Without it, boxers would be like us. Fearful. Weak. Sensible. Human. They wouldn't do what they do.

Back in Hammersmith, George Groves lets his coach, Shane McGuigan, wrap his hands before cruising through eight rounds of sparring with two light-heavyweights, one of whom is a six-fight novice repeatedly tagged by stinging counterpunches throughout. His nose is bloodied but he hangs tough. Afterwards, his coach emphasises he's still learning and therefore shouldn't get disheartened by the painful experience. 'It's all money in the bank,' he says, wiping the twenty-one-year-old's nose with a towel. By 'money', he means the rounds, the experience, not necessarily the hurtful punches, but, in boxing, it all amounts to the same thing. Pain is experience. Pain is money.

Groves, the teacher, sifts through a sports bag for a dry change of clothes and then reappears beside me as I stand by the door. 'How did the people you interviewed react to what happened to them?' he asks more or less out of the blue, possibly now relieved and liberated by the fact the day's fighting is over. That or he's just genuinely interested. Certainly, it can no longer be disregarded as small talk. Quite the opposite. I detect from his tone and the serious expression on his sweat-drenched face that my answer is somehow important to him and that this taboo subject is one he can handle because he is now mature and wise, has won and lost big fights, has been hurt and done the hurting and is, at twenty-eight, comfortable with the cold, hard truths of his profession. Long gone is the kid reprimanded by Chris Eubank for dropping his guard all those years ago.

'Pretty much every single one of them were never the same,' I finally say, 'either in terms of their boxing career or personal life. Barry McGuigan is one of the few exceptions. He was still able to go on and achieve.'

George knows all about Barry. He's now coached by his son. It's the others he wants to know more about. Revealing, too, that his fascination is rooted in the journey of the survivors, those who have to live with the guilt, as opposed to the demise of the victim. It firms up the notion that a boxer's great fear, greater even than being injured or killed in the ring, is being fingered as the one who cut short the life of someone else. 'When you spoke to them, did they all react the same way?' he says. 'You know, when they told you their story.'

DOG ROUNDS

Drunk on this unexpected interest, I tell him about Gabriel Ruelas and his death wish, I tell him about Raúl Hirales and his therapy sessions in Mexico, and I even tell him about James Crayton and his reconstruction of the right hand used to end the life of Johnny Montantes in a Vegas hotel ballroom. We then leave the gym and talk about something else. Purer things, like fatherhood; George recently became a dad for the first time to a boy named Teddy. He tells me what it's like and explains how it has changed his perspective on life, on what is important and what is not. He offers an insight, a small window into his new world, but never any more than that. Perhaps he doesn't want to scare me off.

It's my turn. I'm back at Wembley Arena eight months after Nick Blackwell collapsed here and I stood and watched. Little has changed. It's still pathetically sterile and half-empty, the boxing ring shoved towards the far end of the arena like an unruly child banished to the naughty step, and the majority of the 2,500 present are high on a concoction of alcohol, drugs and impending violence. Some combine the three. I'm here solely for the violence. It's served in generous portions, too, just as it was in March, only this time we will get a full thirty-six minutes' worth, because George Groves, competing in his twenty-eighth professional fight, experiences such a pain in his swollen right hand – the fist used to punish – that he is unable to finish cherry-picked German-based Kazakh Eduard Gutknecht in the allotted time. Mismatched on paper and then in reality, Groves does everything but stop Gutknecht. He pounds him to the body, rocks him to his boots and blows up his eye with his shotgun jab, causing it to gradually close and dominate his face. Yet still there is no climax. Not even an anti-climax, one produced by a ringside doctor, as witnessed in March. That would be preferable to this, I start to think. This slow, repetitive, pointless torture.

The sounds bring back the worst kind of memories. The sounds of the punches – thudding, whipping, crunching – and the sounds of the righteous oracles to my left and right and behind me. The horrified gasps, the dramatic oohs and aahs, the moments of surprising foresight that emerge through a haze of beer and cocaine.

'Look at the state of his face.'

'The geezer needs to be stopped. He's got nothing left.'

'His fucking trainer's got the towel in his hand but ain't doing anything.'

'He's got his hands up protecting himself but he's just looking to survive.'

'He looks like the bloke from *The Goonies*.'

Gutknecht hears the final bell, a moral victory of sorts, and we all go home. All apart from Eduard Gutknecht, that is. He will soon complain he feels unwell and collapse in his changing room. He will then be taken to St Mary's Hospital in Paddington, the same hospital in which Nick Blackwell was treated earlier in the year, as news of his deteriorating condition reaches the rest of us in cars and taxis and trains at around midnight. For some, drug-addled or not, the information has a sobering effect. There is talk of a brain bleed, sedation, operation, coma, and the inevitable backlash begins. Should've been pulled out after ten rounds, they say. Had nothing left. What was the corner thinking? Not another one.

Groves keeps a low profile and waits for news. He remembers the conversation we had a week ago. It plays on his mind. It unnerves him. When we communicate the next day, the Saturday, he mentions the conversation, the eeriness of it, its tempting of fate, before signing off with, 'Scary old game, this boxing malarkey.'

He saw for himself.

It seems only fitting to end a book about guilt with one final confession. Yet the guilt which follows this particular confession weighs heavier than the guilt I felt when returning to ringside just weeks after seeing a boxer in a coma, or indeed the guilt I felt when secretly urging professional wrestlers to do away with child-friendly theatrics and actually punch each other in Mexico City. The guilt is greater, also, than the guilt I feel every time I set eyes on the cover image of this book, one of Duk Koo Kim inert on the ring canvas, and visualise an embittered Ray 'Boom Boom' Mancini calling me a hypocritical piece of shit the next time I see him.

He's right. I probably am a hypocrite. A liar, too. When I said George Groves was the first and only active boxer with whom I had a conversation regarding the finer details of this book, I was, in the tradition of all who inhabit the sport – promoters, managers and fighters – telling only a half-truth. There had, in fact, been another boxer. This one, the one before Groves, had been an active boxer when I started writing the book, but, by the time it was finished, so too was he. He had retired. Call it poetic licence, then, that I initially claimed someone else had been the first. Better yet, call it the very thing fighters, the world over, use to seduce you when formulating grudge matches in order to sell pay-per-view events. Call it bullshit.

'What's it about?' asked Nick Blackwell in Aldershot the day he felt fat and hankered for something sweet upon finishing his coffee.

He meant the book. I told him.

'Heavy stuff,' he replied.

THE END

'I know. You can imagine what it was like watching your fight in March...'

'Yeah, of course. So I get a mention, yeah?'

'Had to,' I said. 'You'll be pleased to know you are my happy ending.'

Blackwell laughed. 'Wicked.'

'Do you want to read it? I kind of think you should.'

'I'll read it when it comes out.'

Too soon, I thought. Maybe that was why. 'I could just send you the bits about you and about the recovery.'

'No, honestly, I'd rather buy myself a copy and read it on holiday. Give me something to look forward to. Don't spoil it for me.'

If only I had.

On 26 November, a Saturday night, eight days after Eduard Gutknecht was placed in an induced coma, the news broke. The news nobody expected and only a few feared. Nick Blackwell had earlier that week, on the Tuesday, decided to engage in a sparring session with Hasan Karkardi, a licensed professional light-heavyweight, at a boxing club in Devizes, Wiltshire. Punches were thrown, heads were hit. You know where the story goes from here. It was a move so misguided it returned Nick, the one who got away, to a coma, only this time he required emergency surgery to remove part of his skull due to the swelling on his brain. The initial prognosis was bleak. Friends and family, all of whom had barely recovered from the drama of March, worried he'd be paralysed if he ever woke. Doctors prepared them for the worst. It was different this time round. They all knew it. Hope was in short supply. Eight months on from the first coma, inquisitions replaced donations and anger replaced sympathy. How could he be so foolish? How could he be so selfish? There was a feeling he'd cheated his second chance at life. How dare he. Poor Mike Towell was never afforded the same opportunity.

But if there's one thing I know, based on the experience of writing this book, it's that Nick Blackwell didn't decide to spar again because he's stupid or ungrateful or because he didn't value his second chance. Nor was his rash, life-altering decision sparked by an inherent rebellious streak or because he was struggling to adapt to civilian life. No, as far as I can see, Nick Blackwell sparred again for one simple yet tragic reason: he was addicted to fighting. It was a habit he couldn't kick.

Consider the evidence. He applied for a trainer's licence not because he had immediate plans to train fighters but because he just wanted to stay close. He wanted to linger. Be in corners, be around gyms, still be involved. Remain relevant. Furthermore, in this domain, his comfort zone, he was labelled a miracle man and peers were quick to compliment him on his recovery. Same old Nick, they said. You'd never know he came so close to dying. And yet, unbeknown to these well-wishers, the more this survival story was perpetuated, the more Nick's hope grew, the more he was inclined to disregard his newfound vulnerability and the more he yearned to be hit around the head again.

He also came to realise the following painful truths: surfing, though he loved it, wasn't fighting; reading, though he wanted to try it, wasn't fighting; opening a gym, though part of his plan, wasn't fighting. And every time he passed a mirror and detected his face had softened or sat down and felt his belly roll over the top of his shorts, Nick knew the only way to feel fit again, feel himself again, was to revert to type. He *needed* to box. It was the thing that defined him. The thing that completed him. Mirrors, he told himself, were for shadowboxing not introspection.

THE END

Retrospection, meanwhile, prompts me to say this: Nick Blackwell probably recovered *too* well. He was *too* able. Able to move, able to leap from rocks, able to train, able, in his mind, to compete. As a consequence, he got comfortable, complacent. As did we. We took him for granted. When he alluded to a rematch with Chris Eubank Jr, it was fine to laugh because it was said in jest, his tongue lodged firmly in his cheek. It was gallows humour. He was taking the piss. You know, being Nick. By the same token, when playfully sparring his brother, or the men and women with whom I watched him move around in Aldershot, it was deemed okay because it was harnessed and under control. But whose control? Nick's control. Nick said it was okay.

Nick said. Nick thought. Nick believed. We must surely now know too much trust and power was placed in the destructive hands and confused mind of a young man who knew nothing else but to fight; a young man whose default setting was the very thing that damaged him; a young man who pointedly refused to read anything from this book not because he assumed it would suck or because its subject matter was too raw but, in actual fact, because he concluded he was healthy enough to one day box again and to do so, to make this dream a reality, he needed to distance himself from all logical thinking and the worst-case scenario and instead embrace a necessary delusion.

In essence, this book would have been his voice of reason and a man in the throes of addiction has no use for a pamphlet preaching the virtues of rehab. Because boxers, like addicts, lie constantly to themselves and those around them. They lie to sell fights. They lie when they say they want to fight the best. They convince themselves and others that training camp has been their greatest to date when aware the truth is quite the opposite. They lie in order to make sense of the very thing they do for a living. They tell themselves they won't get hurt. They claim they don't get nervous. That they're never scared. That they don't feel pain. All lies, all said for self-preservation, but perfectly acceptable within the parameters of the fight game.

Which is precisely why I believed Nick Blackwell when he told me he was done with boxing and that his initial injury had somehow been a blessing in disguise. I shared his optimism and his dream of moving on and leading a normal life. I stayed on script. When he called boxing a 'mug's game', I bought it. Maybe I *wanted* to hear it. I even said he'd found salvation. *Salvation.* Who was the mug now? I trusted the words of a professional boxer – a breed of men and women for whom dishonesty is a prerequisite of their trade – and chose to do so because it made my task so much easier. Awkward conversations were swerved. Painful images were wiped clean. Nick was back to his best. Better than before, in fact. Now he could move on, which meant I could do the same, and so could everyone else. He was my happy ending.

Yet, regrettably, while we all moved on, the temptation of the fight game, the addiction, stuck around.

The Blackwell family had to wait until the Thursday before Christmas to see Nick emerge from his second coma of the year. A 'Christmas miracle' they called it. For Nick, it was The Start. A new one. Another one. An uncertain one. The start of rehabilitation, much longer this time, and the start of his Plan C, whatever that might be.

For me, it was The End. Heard enough, seen enough. 'Boom Boom' Mancini had warned me the day would come: 'Napoleon said that after the age of thirty a man's spirit is not made for war. He meant your values change, your ideology changes, everything changes.'

ACKNOWLEDGEMENTS

I've been lucky enough to interview many fighters over the years. Some you remember, some you're quick to forget. But each of the men interviewed for this book will unquestionably stay with me. They will stay with me because they shared stories they hadn't shared with other people. They will stay with me because I saw them cry and heard their voices crack. Most of all, though, they will stay with me because their honesty and integrity restored my faith in a sport that today overflows with hype men and chancers more often than not faking it for a pay-per-view hit.

For making me believe in boxers again, I want to thank, in order of appearance, George Khalid Jones, Hamilton 'Rocky' Kelly (as well as Harry and John Holland), Ray 'Boom Boom' Mancini, Gabriel Ruelas, James 'Too Sweet' Crayton (and referee Kenny Bayless), Raúl Hirales (and translator Tom Thorogood), Al Seeger, Barry McGuigan and Richie Wenton, all of whom are featured in this book. I'd also like to thank Colin Lake, Jesús Chávez, Teon Kennedy and Steve Dotse, whose stories, in the end, shaped my thought process rather than the book itself.

Dog Rounds, in its original form, made no mention of Nick Blackwell, the Eubank family or George Groves. That it now does saddens me because it means they were all involved in events, during the course of me writing the book, which suddenly made them relevant to the story I was trying to write, one told from my perspective. It's also a reminder that I found myself too close to something I now know can only be enjoyed – *truly enjoyed* – from afar. Even so, I want to acknowledge them. Their actions and words educated me. They changed me.

On a lighter note, I'd like to thank a couple of authors. The first, Donald McRae, has been an invaluable source of advice over the years, but never more so than on the day I told him about a book I had gone away and written on the quiet. By now accustomed to seeing my ideas fester on hard drives rather than bookshelves, I was prepared, I told him, to self-publish an e-book or email it the way of any rinky-dink publisher kind enough to throw me a bone (or book deal). But he told me to have some belief. He said the idea was strong. He pointed me in the right direction. 'Let me know how you get on,' he said. So I did.

The second author, Paul Beatty, was someone I met at Goldsmiths University in late 2016, shortly after he'd won the Man Booker Prize for *The Sellout*. This was no prearranged meet-up, nor were we alone; there were many others present, all as engaged as I was when Paul discussed his brilliant book, all as keen to get their copy signed as I was, all as impatient in the queue as I was. But a conversation I had with Paul was

ACKNOWLEDGEMENTS

personal to me and motivated and inspired me in such a way that it deserves a note of appreciation.

He first wondered if I was studying at the university. I said 'no'. He then asked if I was in the process of writing anything, to which I replied, sheepishly, I was finishing a book. 'What's it about?' he asked. I explained. My response prompted him to close my copy of his book, grab a post-it note from nearby and begin scribbling down the address of his home in New York. 'Man, you have got to send that to me,' he said. 'It sounds great.'

For the next ten minutes I held up the line and Paul, riffing on boxing, clearly a passion of his, forgot all about signing my book and those of the people behind me. 'No shit,' he said. 'Barry McGuigan? I didn't know that.' Few do, Paul, few do. He eventually signed my book. 'Now make sure you send me *your* book,' he said. 'I need to read it.' So I did.

Another memorable moment in the process of writing *Dog Rounds* occurred in early-2017, at Megan's cafe on the Kings Road, when Matt Phillips, the book's editor, sat opposite me and asked a question: 'Why did you write this book?'

Taken out of context, the question could be deemed an insult. He'd just finished reading the first draft and this was hardly a glowing appraisal. But he'd also shown an interest in the book within minutes of me telling him about it, made a habit of buying me coconut cappuccinos – top ten in London, apparently – and was, I soon realised, precisely the editor I needed. Basically, he made me ask questions of myself I probably didn't want to ask. For that, I owe him a huge debt of gratitude. I'd like to extend that thanks to his colleagues at Blink as well, particularly Oliver Holden-Rea, Lizzie Dorney-Kingdom, September Withers and Justine Taylor.

Finally, a big thank you to my parents (for just about everything), and to my wife, Louisa, my number one reader and cheerleader, someone whose commitment, both to our relationship and the cause, was cemented the moment she gleefully accompanied me on a day trip to a boxing gym during week two of our Mexico honeymoon. That's true love, I'm told.